GOING THE

DISTANCE

The Journey of a Vasculitis Patient on
the road to Olympic Glory

Brandon Hudgins

With John Fries

Contents

This book wouldn't have been possible without the support and encouragement of Team Brandon. This book is for you!

Foreword

By Chris Moen

In the summer of 2013, Brandon and I decided to live together in Boone, North Carolina and train for the 2016 Track and Field Olympic Trials. I had just graduated college at Appalachian State University in Boone, and like Brandon was seeking to postpone adulthood and chase life as a professional distance runner. Brandon, on the other hand, had just completed his 4th and final round of chemotherapy. It was his second relapse with his Vasculitis disorder Granulomatosis with Polyangiitis since his diagnosis on April 25th 2008.

At the time, I knew Brandon as a friend. Someone who had similar talents to me as a runner and someone who had the same goals and aspirations. Our friendship dated back to 2009 when Brandon entered Appalachian State's graduate school with 2 years of his collegiate track eligibility remaining. When I heard Brandon was transferring to Appalachian, his story was told by our coach Mike Curcio a little like this:

"So there is this guy who ran 3:49 for 1500 meters (equivalent to a 4:06 mile) as a sophomore at Winthrop University. He has been battling a strange autoimmune disease, but he's got 2 years of eligibility left and wants to join the team. Because of his disease he hasn't been able to run competitively for a while, but he is healthy and going to give it a shot again"

3:49 was better than any App runner at the time, thus making him an anomaly to our team. I remember meeting him for the first time while he was on a visit. He showed up looking like he came straight from a Guns n' Roses Concert. He had on slick shades, a rockstar haircut, skinny black jeans and a black leather jacket. It was April, and if it were raining I don't think he would've taken the shades off. But he didn't come across as a tough guy. He was nice, and I sensed that his appearance gave him a bit of comfort. Some people can just pull it off, and Brandon seemed to have that aura solidified. In a strange way I think it gave him a feeling of acceptance while keeping a safe distance from intimate tragedy. But then again, maybe it's just rock n roll.

From that time on we became good friends and teammates, but it wasn't until we lived together that Brandon and I became best friends. It was in those years that I got to know the pages of this book in great detail. It was in those years that we ran countless miles together and had countless late night conversations that could take any direction. To know the basic accounts of Brandon's life is one thing, but to hear the detail and see the blood, sweat, and tears that went into his endeavors as an athlete and human being is enamoring.

As I noted, our goal in 2013 was to make the Olympic Trials. I came short of that goal; falling out of love with running and spending the upcoming Olympic year washing dishes and failing to land all but one kickflip on a skateboard. I still lived in Boone and I even worked at the same resort that Brandon worked at as a front desk employee while he trained for the Olympic Trials. I saw Brandon's trials and tribulations, which were centered around an ultimate goal. Seeing him work the desk job while training without a sponsor or a team really put his work ethic into perspective. In track especially, you need the right people in your corner to get you into good races and good scenarios to be successful. All through 2016 Brandon was the scrapper that always had to push his way through the door. It was clear to me that Brandon's motivation was and always has been self driven. He was able to break through that door and solidify his spot in the Olympic Trials in a race at Furman University on June 4th with a time of 3:38.20. Getting this opportunity required not only years of training but years of persistence to build a strong reputation to even get the opportunity to run in a race of this caliber. This race was only 1 of 3 opportunities in the country that Brandon would have to achieve his qualifying mark that summer, fortunately he nailed it on the first attempt.

When it became 100% certain that Brandon had in fact qualified for the Trials, I bought a plane ticket to join him in Eugene, Oregon. I had no idea that I could fall out of love with running only to be one of its biggest fans at the Olympic Trials. The irony was quite poetic for me and speaks at large to Brandon's story. When I got to the Eugene airport I noticed Olympic Trials promotional advertisements everywhere. They were all the same and the slogan was "The Heroes are coming to TrackTown!" or something of that nature. With this slogan was a basic graphic of a male and female track athlete. They looked like video game characters or boring action figure characters that could have shown up had you Google image searched "generic track athlete animation." I found it patronizing to call these track athletes heroes and place a nameless faceless animation to the slogan. It reminded me of Brandon's intimate story and how unpublicized and unappreciated it truly was. It reminded me how he had to pay for his plane ticket and place to stay for those 10 days. Even a $30 entry fee to race, and in return his only physical prize was an Olympic Trials coffee mug. But as the trials ended and the excitement settled, I could only smile as I flew back home looking at these advertisements. All along Brandon has been living out the journey of a true hero as illustrated by Joseph Campbell. From having a true *"call to adventure"* to "approaching the inmost cave" of mental and emotional conflict to conquering his goal and "seizing the sword." This is a story not just for runners or those with a rare disease, but anybody who has ever wanted something regardless of the obstacles in the way.

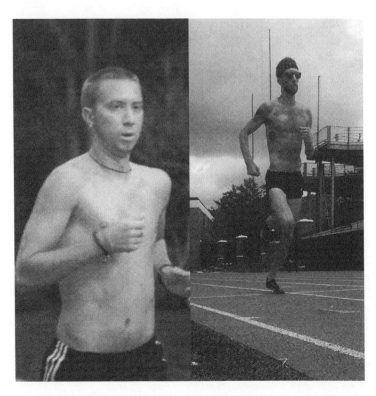

A glimpse at my desire and dedication to my craft. On the left is a picture taken while I was on chemotherapy and loads of other drugs to save my body from Vasculitis in 2008. On the right is a picture from a workout just before breaking 4 minutes in the mile in 2015. The pages that follow describe the physical and mental journey.

Introduction

For better and for worse, I am Brandon Hudgins. I'm a native to South Carolina, a competitive distance runner, and so many other things. I try to be a good son, a good brother, a good boyfriend, and a good friend. I've accomplished what many would describe as wonderful, remarkable and personally fulfilling things in my 30 short years on this Earth. I've traveled across the U.S., met hordes of amazing people, made new friends, been interviewed for national magazines and network television, and competed for a spot on the 2016 U.S. Olympic Team at 1500 meters. What makes my running story so unique is the fact that I also suffer from a rare, autoimmune disease called Vasculitis. More specifically Granulomatosis with Polyangiitis, a disorder that causes inflammation of blood vessels causing granulomas to form in my organs and slowly or rapidly shut them down.

Outside of my insane inner thoughts, the only thing that's truly wrong with my body is that my immune system thinks some of my organs are the enemy. I'm basically allergic to myself - Which is incredibly ironic for a narcissist like myself. My own immune system (my B-cells to be specific) have decided to go haywire since the fall of 2007. I was diagnosed at age 21 after suffering for over 6 months from major health problems such as joint pain, breathing problems, hearing loss, extreme fatigue, sinus infections, bloody noses, night sweats, circulation problems and nearly losing my kidneys. As of the writing of this book in 2017, there is no known cause or cure for my disease. Until medicine and science can find a cure, I will live with the disease for the rest of my life. I've been lucky enough to achieve remission on several occasions for a few years at a time. Just long enough to live a semi-normal life and chase a silly childhood dream.

The oddest thing is that despite battling my disorder since the age of 21 and having an overwhelming sense of pride in some of the athletic accomplishments I've had in my life, I still feel unfulfilled. In many ways I even feel like a failure. I know I shouldn't feel this way, but I do. I've had time goals and championships in my mind since before I could remember, and quite frankly I've never gotten to the level I thought I could. If my health or circumstances took the sport away from me tomorrow, it would be hard for me to truly be happy with my accomplishments. I feel like if I don't accomplish the goals I've set, then I will always be living with the nagging voice of "what if" in the back of my mind.

Now I work closely with the Vasculitis Foundation, an organization that provides education and support to fellow patients around the world. I've had amazing experiences over the last year and a half working with the Vasculitis community, but at times it's hard for me to get so much praise and support from one group of people like the Vasculitis community, yet still feel like a complete outsider in my own sport. I've climbed the ladder of success in my sport, yet I still don't feel like an insider in my own sport. Maybe it's just my imagination, but either way, it's one of the things that still compels me to chase my dreams in the sport of Track and Field.

I've always felt like the underdog, partly because I always have been. I still feel like the 17-year-old Brandon who got his ass kicked at the South Carolina State Cross-Country Meet and could barely be happy that his own team still won the state title. Or the 18-year-old Brandon who was angry that bigger schools weren't recruiting me out of high school. Or the 19-year-old Brandon that felt like I had to prove all those big schools wrong.

At the time of this writing, I'm 30 years old, unemployed, and chasing a childhood dream that at times seems like a waste of time. Often I stare at myself in the mirror and wonder if what I'm doing is even worth all the energy and struggle I've been through, just to accomplish a few items at the bottom of my bucket list. It's a dangerous thought trap for someone with crippling anxiety. It makes me wonder if what I accomplish will ever be enough to satisfy myself. Who knows? I sure as hell don't. That's why I'm sharing some lessons I've learned on my journey because I have gotten a whiff of what it's like to be at the top, and I can tell you that it's worth it, if what you are doing is truly your passion. The curse of striving for such high standards can be a giant burden on yourself and your loved ones at times. But when you do find those moments—no matter how brief they are—it makes them that much more special.

As you will learn in the pages that follow, I wrote this book for two people: you and me.

While I don't wish or encourage anyone to be just like me, I do want to share my experiences for those who have felt down and want to give you some tools to make your dreams come true. The one thing I have truly learned about myself over the last several years of struggle is that I want to help people. That's what I've realized is my goal beyond anything else in life. I want to encourage people to make their dreams come true. By doing that, maybe I'll be able to see mine come true as well.

I live with extreme regret and worry every day. I'm writing this book because, ultimately, I think my experiences in life have made me an incredibly resilient person and I wish to impart some of my experiences and lessons to give you tools to succeed on your journey.

As I share my story and tips that have helped bring me from the depths of my own mental hell, remember that I have made loads of mistakes and failed myself and others almost every step of the way. That's life though. How we pick up the pieces and move forward determines who we are as people. If some of the idiotic mistakes I've made, the dark times I've gone through and the lessons

I've learned can provide you with enough inspiration and motivation to get you out of your rut and inspire you to achieve something for yourself, then this shit show I call a life will have some meaning.

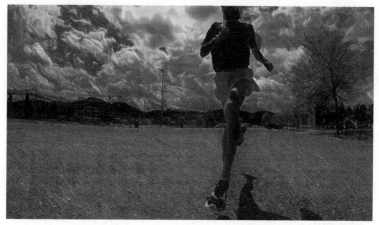

Fire in the Sky by Bill Wilde

All Hope is Gone

Life has a way of yanking the rug out from under us and causing us to lose our balance. You never know when these events might strike. Sometimes it's as you are trying to leave the old house and move on with life. Other times, it's as you walk into the new house and thought you were all settled in.

It's unavoidable. Life will eventually catch up to you. We all carry trauma from our past experiences. It's a part of growing up. Some of us experience it young and often, while others get lucky and make it to adulthood without many traumatic events. Either way, life's trauma is inescapable.

I've lived through a lot of traumatic experiences in my life. My family lost a beautiful girl at just 19 days old when I was 4 years old. I lost two running teammates before the age of 15, and at 21 years old was diagnosed with a rare Vasculitis disorder that affects roughly one or two people per million. So by my mid twenties I was already carrying a 747 aircraft full of traumatic experiences around. Believe it or not the event that seemingly wrecked my emotional stability and caused me to finally fall on my back helplessly was experiencing my first panic attack. By age 26 I had been hit so hard by life while trying to stay on my feet, that my mind finally failed me. Being a type A person, I was probably predisposed to this condition anyway, but by 26 my mind had finally had enough. My old way of thinking and processing emotion no longer worked.

Through so many of the difficult experiences in my early life, I somehow managed to get back on my feet and find my center. You may be wondering what I mean by center. When you are centered as a person you have confidence in yourself to handle the challenges of life. You are aware of yourself and your actions. You are a conscious decision maker. Your actions in life lead directly towards your plan or goals in life. Early in life fighting to keep my center came naturally somehow. No matter what life seemed to throw at me I was able to pick myself up and move forward with intent and purpose.

For instance, fighting my rare disease was just like training for a big season or race. I just kept my head down and fought hard for what I wanted in life. I was great at it. But fighting anxiety and panic attacks completely blew a new rut through my mind. To learn that my strong willed mind was fighting back was the yank of the rug that landed me on my back and unable to find a way up. It was an invisible enemy, one that was inside my own mind. After being diagnosed with anxiety and panic attacks, it was unsettling to learn that I was going to have to reprogram my brain to be myself. I could no longer hold onto the anger and aggression that had driven me for so many years. I was going to have to learn to let things go and take a more low key mental approach, or I would keep ending up in the hospital.

As they say, the first step in understanding is recognition. I had a hard time wrapping my brain around all this. First, a rare disease. Now my own mind, which had always been my friend, was attacking me. How was I ever going to win if I couldn't trust my own mind?

The author, Pema Chodron, was recommended to me by a dear friend who had also lost herself. Looking back, it was interesting that she never recommended a specific book, only the name of an author, which was brilliant. I was able to search through Pema's work and find the title that lept out at me. If you're not familiar with her, Pema is an American Tibetan Buddhist who has written several books.

Through her misfortunes in life she was able to learn to let go and then teach others how to heal. Her book When Things Fall Apart showed me I already had the necessary tools to conquer my new challenges. She introduced me to the idea of hopelessness. Now, I realize that that term can sound depressing to people who don't really understand it. Humans waste a lot of good energy on hope. The definition of hope is *an expectation or desire for a certain outcome*, when often we have no control over the outcomes of situations in life.

The feeling of hopelessness for many comes when life beats them down to the point they think they can't continue. Life can smack you in the face with so many different forms of adversity to knock you down—a lost job, death of a loved one, divorce, health issues, money problems, drug problems, etc. —it's great to reflect and learn what's important in life. These are times to grow, and often we must fail before we can learn. So many of us are hardheaded and stubborn and refuse to learn until we are faced with a difficult ultimatum.

When I was reading Pema's book, she often spoke of the feeling of groundlessness. It's that feeling you get when your head is spinning, you don't know which way to reach to catch yourself. All you know is that you feel out of control and on a crash course for rock bottom, where you're going to land flat on your back. The question then becomes, what do I do?

Who we are in life is determined by how we react when we lose our balance. I'd be lying if I said I always handled it properly because the reality is that I've failed many times, and will fail again. The biggest lesson I've learned that I can pass on to anyone struggling with groundlessness, or feeling like his or her life is in the eye of a hurricane, is to find your center. What does that mean?

Learn to sit still and let things move through you and around you.
Learn what needs your immediate attention and what can wait.
Learn what to fight for, and what you need to let go of.
Learn to be ok with failure.
Learn to be happy with the pursuit.

These are all clichés we have all heard or read, but they have been repeated over and over for a reason:

They are true.

I have the phrase "All Hope is Gone" adorned with roses tattooed across my chest. For me all hope is gone means learning to find happiness in the pursuit and accept the outcome. All the hope in the world won't get you the things you want in life. You have to find your center, work to keep your balance, and accept that you will not always get what you want or deserve. My tattoo is a reminder of all the hard times I've been through in life and been able to find my way back.

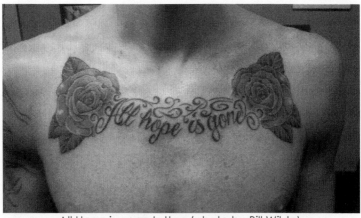

All Hope is gone tattoo (photo by Bill Wilde)

Not knowing what lies on the other side of a tragedy can be scary for many people, myself included. But you have to embrace that change and take that step to get out of your comfort zone or you will probably never be able to chase your true dreams. All hope is gone means that you have to be willing to accept the fact that you may fail, but still be happy with your journey and struggles, no matter the outcome. As an ancient Chinese philosopher once said, "The journey is the reward." Change also helps you learn to find your center and your balance during the most chaotic times in your life. You must become the eye of the storm. Be the calm that is in the center of the storm, or the storm will sweep you away. If you are like me, you have found yourself off balance more than a few times in your life. When I didn't find my way, my mind and actions lead me down a path of drugs, alcohol and destructive behavior. It becomes a high speed highway into the dark pits of the human mind and spirit.

At this point in time I seem to have found my center, but several times over the last 10 years, I've completely lost myself to the tides of the storm and visited some disturbing places. This hasn't just been tough for me, but also tough on my loved ones. That's one of the shitty things about having a rare disease and also being a self-centered ass at times, it can cause a tremendous amount of pain for your support system. I didn't always recognize the steps that lead me off course, but once I reached the bottom I finally admitted to myself that I needed help. At the bottom my mistakes began to unravel the dream of Olympic glory I was chasing.

As I mentioned in the intro, I am a professional or semi professional distance runner. It has been a goal of mine since I was in high school. I have dreamed of Olympic glory since watching the Olympic Games in the summer of 2004. For U.S. distance runners there are National Championships every summer and an Olympic Trials once every four years. We only have a few chances each year to shine as an athlete on a National stage like most professional athletes. Back in the summer of 2014, I found my dream of being a professional athlete slowly fading. After missing out on the USA Championships once again in June that year, I found myself living in total disarray. I had focused too much on work and running and not given the necessary attention to other parts of my life. I moved into the most disgusting dump I've ever lived in. The one room apartment was up a steep driveway down a nice mountain road. One morning I was running late for work because my workout session had taken longer than expected that morning. Backing out, I flipped my 1995 Toyota 4Runner down the side of my driveway and into that lovely mountain road. Because of the stress I was putting on myself to perform on the track, the stress I was under working a job that was solely to support my running, and trying to also maintain a long distance relationship, had put me at my whits end. It's hard looking back to figure out what I was thinking, but I was really just swept up in my own ego and expected certain things to work out.

When they didn't I got frustrated and let it all get to me. Instead of working methodically to change my circumstances, I had become a victim of them. All of this had led to a lack of sleep, frustrated living circumstances, and horrible training because I was beginning to struggle with my anxiety and depression again. I was less than a year past my new diagnosis and hadn't yet developed the skills to deal with them. As I mentioned before, when things begin to get in the way of my dream-chasing as a runner, I get really worked up, angry and vengeful. This stress has manifested itself into my body to where I had nagging injuries, horrible training sessions, a body that is just worn out. Not a recipe that was going to lead me to the starting line at the Olympic Trials in two years time, but a step I needed to take on my journey.

This is one of the funniest points in my life, and honestly is only fitting to how my life so often plays out. Despite all of this chaos and stress, just two days after flipping my car, I managed to run one of the happiest races I'd had in nearly 2 years. The Liberty Road Mile in Pittsburgh, PA became my savior in a way. After a rough year on the track, being back in the pack of elite milers reminded me that I belonged there. Despite a horrible build up in training for the event for nearly a month, the lack of sleep and wrecking my car two days before the race, I was able to kick with some of the best milers in the country. Now I got my head beat in over the final 100 meters of the race, but I had fought and felt like I belonged again, which was just the spark that I needed.

This made me laugh. Initially, I was angry because I had a great opportunity to finish fourth behind three of the best middle-distance runners in the country. But then I realized how much shit I had put up with in the last few weeks and I laughed, because I knew that if I had been fresh and better prepared it would have been a different race. Another beautiful thing was that I ran without fear for the first time all season and was completely caught up in the amazing atmosphere that the people at Bring Back the Mile and the Liberty Mile put together. I lined up not knowing what my body could handle, but I didn't care--I was going to help put on the show. I was going to dish out whatever my body could handle and I was happy with what I was able to accomplish because so many days during that time period I wondered if all the work was worth it, if I'd ever really get to my goal in 2016, or if I should just throw in the towel. I wanted so badly to end my season, but I kept plugging away and when I least expected it, found my spark. It's also why I continue to make the Liberty Mile a stop on my racing calendar every year. It's a friendly reminder of a terrible time in my life where I found a spark I so desperately needed.

No matter how far off course or deep-in you find yourself (it's pretty bad having to find a new place to live and a new car all in the same week), you have to try and find your center of peace in the chaos. Realizing that there is no cause for all of the bad things and no one to blame will help you release those demons and find that peace with whatever shitstorm life wants to blow your way.

I wasted a lot of my youth and young adulthood hoping for good things to happen to me, and when they didn't, I became angry and bitter at the world around me. This anger and bitterness helped drive me at times, but that fire isn't sustainable. Once that flame burned out I was left empty and cold. I had to find a good log to toss on the burning embers. I learned that if I was going to continue to chase my dream of Olympic glory as a track and field athlete, then I was going to have to be okay with failure. My journey became my purpose.

When people see my All Hope is Gone tattoo they are often caught off guard and surprised. They don't expect someone like me to have such "depressing" words scribbled on my chest. What they don't understand is the power that I have because the hope is gone. After I got the tattoo, I initially loved seeing the reaction and shock on people's faces when they realized what the words said. It gave me a sick pleasure because I've always liked to make people and strangers a little uncomfortable to break down their guard. It's a weird game I picked up somewhere along the way. Maybe it was the years of wearing short shorts in public, getting picked on by my peers, or trying to make up for not fitting in, whatever the case, it's been a hobby of mine for a long time. Now it's no longer a weird game I get some sick pleasure from, but a chance to for me to share something about my vasculitis journey. As a Vasculitis Ambassador for the Vasculitis Foundation, it's my goal to use every opportunity to share, not just for my sake, but for all vasculitis patients around the world.

Vasculitis hasn't just forced me to change my outlook on life or the way I live, it's changed so much of who I am as a person. All hope is gone is a great example of that. Without the struggle, it would be impossible for me to understand my current life position. Sharing my experiences is a chance for me to explain to people that as someone living with a rare, potentially fatal disease, I can't sit around wishing and hoping for the things I want in life to happen. If that were true, I'd never get out of bed in the morning. I'd spend most of my time hoping for a cure. That would rob me of all my energy. I've watched hope destroy people and hold them down. I realize that it can sound insensitive and mean to say that spending time hoping is wasteful, but it's how I feel and a lesson I think many people could use to empower themselves. That's why I'm sharing so much of my journey with people. I've had it rough, and learned an awful lot from my mistakes and misfortunes.

There are still times I lay awake in bed at night wondering if this has all been some sick twisted dream I've been living the last 10 years. When I find myself doing that, it can become very toxic for my energy and progress. It's one of the things that can cause any person living with an incurable disease to go absolutely crazy. I watched my parents struggle with the loss of one child and the questioning of why her and our family. Then again when my vasculitis struck, wondering why it could happen to such a "healthy" young, good person, like me. I've seen too many people get consumed by those thoughts and questions. After dealing with those thoughts so often, I realized that I couldn't live my life that way wishing, hoping, and wondering, what if? That's why Pema's words were so powerful for me at so many different parts of my journey.

People assume that because I no longer have hope that I have nothing to live for. On the contrary. Now, because I don't have hope, it means I no longer allow that desire to rule my life or my happiness. The reality is, every time that my vasculitis strikes, I have a brush with death and there is a chance that it may be the one that ends my journey. I can't get tied up in the outcome. I have goals that I am working hard towards, but I also realize that I may never get the chance to reach them. I've been fortunate enough so far to still accomplish some of those goals like a sub 4 minute mile and qualifying for the Olympic Trials, but I have life goals way beyond an athletic career. My journey now has brought me the ability to help others along the way because of my personal struggles, and that has added another giant log to the fire raging in the pit of my stomach to leave my mark on this world while I can.

At this point, my journey has transcended anything that I could want. It has become less about me and more about inspiring others, like yourself. That was a much larger goal than I could ever have imagined five or six years ago and, quite frankly, something that I couldn't have handled until I had found my bottom. But when you work hard, learn from your mistakes and keep moving forward, you learn that you can take on a much bigger load than you would have ever expected you could to carry. That lesson I learned from being a distance runner. As they say life's a marathon and not a sprint. Training for a marathon requires dedication and purpose with every step. Most days are a grind. A lot of the work will be put in when others aren't watching, but when you get that moment to shine on race day or on your life journey, all the hard long work will pay off.

In sharing my story and working with the Vasculitis Foundation to promote Vasculitis Awareness, I have had so many people tell me that I have given them hope. My response is always the same, "I don't want to give you hope in your tough situations, I want to give you inspiration." As much as this pains me to say, it's very similar to the old wise tale: You don't just give a man a fish; you teach him how to fish, and that's my goal. By giving inspiration instead of hope, I want to give the tools to succeed in your journey. Inspiration can help you find your desires.

If my misfortunes can help someone on his or her journey—you, perhaps—it's a win for both of us. It gives my struggles greater meaning and purpose, while also helping someone on a journey. We are helping each other. Recently the joy that helping others has given me has made some recent struggles more bearable. The pressure may get to me at times, but this time around I know where my eye of the storm lies. I haven't fallen off the ledge, gotten swept up in the negativity storm, or given into my destructive thoughts and behaviors. So ultimately these interactions are important for both of us when I can connect on a personal level, and then in turn that person can be inspired by my journey. Like I said before, the why matters so much.

I know I will have many more battles to fight on my journey—some that I probably can't even fathom yet, I'm sure. For all I know, I may not have even found my rock bottom. But the uncertainty in life is a lot less scary with the right tools. One of those is self-help, if you want to find a way to get better, you have to make that decision. That doesn't mean it won't require help, it just means that ultimately you have to be the one that makes the decision to battle. If you have confidence in yourself to find a path no matter the struggle, then you know that you can take on life's greatest challenges.

Right now while writing this book, I am living in one of the most insecure financial positions I have ever been in my adult life. And you know what? I find it incredibly invigorating. Now, I realize that it's not for everyone, but living out your dream on a daily basis with an extreme probability of failure, but with the utmost confidence in yourself is the most fulfilling thing I've done in my life. I'm happier than I ever was with a weekly paycheck. When I made the decision to completely embrace the uncertainty and chase my dream unencumbered, I began to live. Before I was fighting every day for a chance to possibly succeed. Now I live to succeed. My success and my failures are no one's fault but my own. It's truly beautiful.

The Importance of Friends and Support

I've made it this far in my life solely because of my support network. This network includes my family— my mom, dad, brother, sister, and girlfriend—and my immediate friends, who are really like family to me.

If not for this special group of people, I would have given up on life back in 2013. That year I had finally reached the end of my mental rope. I had suffered through my initial battle with my Vasculitis, been healthy for almost 3 years before battling relapses in 2012 and 2013. By mid 2013 I was done fighting. Working so hard to find my groove again only to have the rug yanked out from under me time and time again was just too much for my brain at 26 years old. Factor in some other "regular" life problems, and I just didn't want to fight anymore. But every time I've slipped into depression, let myself slip into dark moments in my head where I just can't see another way out, I've stopped myself from going over the edge only because of my support network.

Cue up some dramatic scene in a million different Hollywood movies where a guy or girl is sitting in a shower crying and wishing they would just die. I'm ashamed to admit this has happened. In those moments it's scary how easy it would be to check out and end the personal suffering. My family and friends are my biggest inspiration, so in the end I couldn't bear the thought of what they would have to go through if I gave in to my self-pity and ended it all. That's really the paradox of depression and suicidal thoughts. You may get relief from your darkness, but your loved ones then take on an even greater pain.

What's so weird is that on the outside, though, it was business as usual. I bragged about being invincible and saying I was going to kick vasculitis's ass again. That's always who I had been, so it was my default response, it was my M.O. and I felt the need to live up to that. Yet secretly on the inside I was screaming for help and couldn't handle the stress of another relapse. This was only the beginning of my high functioning, type A personality finally failing me and crippling me with anxiety and depression. It would be several months before I would learn that I had developed anxiety and depression induced by my struggle with Vasculitis.

To people on the outside, nothing seemed unusual. I got up, went to work and functioned throughout the day. Meanwhile, in my head, I was slowly losing grip with the reality around me. I was looking for ways out of every situation. I hated interacting with people. One of the misconceptions about anxiety and depression is that people assume that depression only means watching a funny movie and not being able to laugh. It wasn't till I finally saw a therapist months later that I realized there are so many varying degrees of anxiety and depression. Since I was still shunning the Vasculitis community at this point, I had no clue that a large majority of Vasculitis (and all rare diseases for that matter) patients struggle with the potentially deadly combo. See I'm a people person by nature. I inherited it from my father who can have hour long conversations with strangers in Wal-Mart. Anytime I was in public or at work, I was really wishing I was home and locked in my room. Even though I hated my living situation, I had found some odd comfort in the isolation of my room. Living barebones trying to make it as a semi professional runner also meant living with no internet or cable TV to save money. So when I went home it was the perfect dungeon to lock myself in mentally and be able to shut out the world and indulge my heinous thoughts.

At that time in 2013 I was living in my hometown of Rock Hill, South Carolina and working as a substitute teacher at my former high school. As I mentioned earlier, I grew up a teacher/coach's kid. Over the 20-plus years of my Dad's education career he has taught or coached a large part of the people in our town. So while I may never know what it's like to be famous on a national scale, being in Rock Hill can be stressful for me. It's very rare that I or any member of my family can go anywhere in town without being stopped or recognized by someone who wants to stop and talk.

Now these are never really bad interactions, but so often they feel gross. People clearly aren't bothering me in the bathroom to get an autograph while I'm trying to take a piss. But when you are suffering silently, these interactions become cumbersome and trying. While this was clearly mostly in my head, I did feel like I was under a microscope anytime I was home in Rock Hill. I've tried time and time again to shove this notion out, knowing full well the power of this community that has been incredibly helpful to my family during tragic times, but I can never shake it.

Because Rock Hill is a smaller town (roughly 70,000 people) in which everybody seemingly knows everybody else, most people there watched as I went through my initial diagnosis and treatment, then a relapse 4 years later. But a second relapse in two years was just too much for the fragile strings of my sanity. It plowed a rut through my mind that I'll likely be navigating the rest of my life (or until science comes through and finds a cure for Vasculitis).

What's so ironic is that my safe haven over the years has become Boone, NC (population 18,000), an even smaller town, but without the family connections to make it seem so small. That's one of the reasons I have loved my isolated town life in Boone. People there don't bother you. They are friendly to interact with, slow paced, and don't look at you in a weird way if you are a little different than them. Actually that's a wrong way of describing it. Everyone in Boone is a little weird and a little different. I wish the same could be said about Rock Hill. Once again I recognize this is probably all just some terrible narrative that I've written in my head, but I've actually had conversations with friends who, like me, have felt the desire to leave. Or maybe that conversation was all in my head too? It's incredibly awkward to feel like an outcast in a community that raised you and has supported your family through thick and thin. But unfortunately it was the reality I had created in my head and the way I often feel going home even today.

Looking back at those joyless days in 2013, it seems overly dramatic and comical at this point, really, but those moments were indeed very real and frightening. I've often tried to describe to people where my mind and body were at during this time and the only word that I can ever seem to find is toxic. My blood was literally toxic from all the drugs I was having to take to keep my immune system in check. My thoughts were toxic with negativity and self pity. My actions were selfish and looking for indulgence. I looked for anything that could ease a few minutes of pain or give me some freedom from my own thoughts. Anything to feel the rush of the athletic and active lifestyle that I missed. When your mind gets warped like this, it takes a concerted effort to start to heal and begin to find yourself again.

Luckily for me, I had some amazing friends in my life who, without realizing it, rescued me from the pit of darkness. When they reached out, I didn't even think, I just jumped.

I moved back to Boone, NC in June of 2013 amid roommate problems and a search for happiness. A friend had gotten me an interview for a valet job parking cars at a resort and offered a couch to sleep on until I could find my own place. On a Thursday in early June of 2013 I drove up to Boone for an interview for a valet position. By Saturday I was back in Boone with all of the belongings I could fit in my 4Runner and used my Master's Degree in Exercise Science to start my new valet job. That summer turned out to be one of the more fascinating summers of my life.

At the time, I was sleeping on my friends' couch till I could figure out my next move in life. No one was really thinking too far ahead. We were all just living and having fun. As a group of friends, none of us knew any different. You put us together in any situation and we would find a way to entertain ourselves. There were five guys living in a small, four-bedroom apartment smack dab in the middle of Boone. We had more friends living in an apartment directly above us and several girls from my Appalachian State cross-country team living just a few doors down in our complex. So that made our complex the hub of fun that summer. There was always something to do: video games to play, adventures to chase, waterfalls to jump off, sports to play, miles to be run, and money to be made. In fact, if the cops had ever ransacked our place, they would have probably been looking for the drugs to go along with all the cash in our apartment. With five guys working service industry jobs that summer, on any given day there were thousands of dollars in $1's and $5's stashed in shoe boxes, the back of drawers and socks. One afternoon, one of my roommates walked out of his room with over $3,000 in small bills from just one week of working four jobs. It truly was comical.

This was exactly what my creeping anxiety and lingering depression needed: things to do. I hadn't learned the skill yet, but the best thing for my anxiety crippled brain was direction or distractions. So if I don't have a direction, I must find ways to distract myself or it's easy to lose control and let the anxiety settle in for a nice stay, which then is a fast track to depression for me. Anybody with anxiety knows that a busy mind needs constant stimulation, ideal time can be dangerous. While the summer was great fun and the much needed change I needed, I was still on the road to suffering my second (still undiagnosed) panic attack. Only now, I was driving 100 mph instead of the 200+ mind warping mph I had previously been driving.

At the time, getting back into running wasn't on my mind. Oh, I had gone out and run with my friends a few times as they trained for the upcoming college or professional season, but I wasn't able to shake that inner feeling of tension in my chest, arms, and mind that I attributed to my vasculitis. So when I went out for runs, I'd try to relax, laugh and enjoy my favorite places to run, but inside I was blowing up. Since my autoimmune disease is based in my vascular system, any time that I have breathing problems or feel like I'm working too hard, I automatically assume it's my vascular system and that my immune system is again attacking my body.

When I moved back to Boone in the summer of 2013, I was just a month removed from four rounds of biological chemotherapy treatment, and by all means, I should have been healing. Well, my body was healing, but my mind still wasn't ready. So as I worked at the resort, hung out with friends and enjoyed my mountain life again, I was trying to figure out my next move. Which is another giant stressor when you feel like you have no direction. When I started applying for coaching jobs at the NCAA level, which had been my initial plan after my competitive running days had ended, the anxiety slowly reared it's ugly head. Luckily after several interviews and the realization that I didn't want to move halfway across the country for a position that paid shit, I sacked that idea and was kind of left to tread water until I could direct my energy elsewhere.

My friends frequently tried to drag me out the door with them for runs. Sometimes I'd say yes, other times I'd say screw it, pop open a beer and cheer them on as they went out the door (no, I'm not the smartest patient in the world, I shouldn't have been drinking or doing some of the other stupid things I did that summer). It probably wasn't a collective effort from all of them, but to them I was BHudg, the guy that had moved up to the mountains in 2009 and joined their team. I was washed up and overweight, yet full of fire to compete again. So they expected no different this time around. They wouldn't let me rest on my laurels apparently. They were expecting more out of me at a time when I was expecting nothing from myself.

You're probably wondering why it's taken me this long to really mention why friends are important, considering this chapter is entitled "The Importance of Friends and Support." Well, my friends changed my direction in life on August 17th, 2013.

On that day, I met several of the Appalachian State team runners and my close friends Chris Moen and Cameron Bean (aka Cameron CronCity Magnum Bean) who were both training as professional runners with the Zap Fitness organization that trains in the Boone area, for a run alongside the Watauga River. It wasn't supposed to be anything special or meaningful. Just another run in a summer filled with runs where I struggled to keep pace with my friends, feel sluggish and closed off and honestly look like a shell of the athlete that I once was. Watauga River Road is a mostly gravel road that has some of the best sweeping views of any run on the East Coast. During my college days at Appalachian State University, it was one of my favorite places to run, but it was about to take on a whole new meaning in my life.

During that run, I ran free for the first time in months! I couldn't believe it. Something just happened. I didn't know it at the time, but in each of my comebacks after flare ups with my Vasculitis, one day for some reason stuff will inexplicably click. After months of toying around with running, feeling like I'd never do it again, not feeling normal, and suffering from severe and crippling anxiety and panic attacks that had finally been diagnosed, I found my happy place on that run. I felt like a runner again. The bug bit me and it bit me hard. That day I didn't feel the tightness in my chest, only the acid pumping through my veins and lead in my legs of a hard effort earned through a fast pace.

Now I'm not one to believe in any sort of fate or destiny, but had that day not happened like it did, I wouldn't have started comeback number three that finally lead me under my lifetime goal of breaking four minutes in the mile in 2015, or qualified for the Olympic Trials in 2016. Which means I wouldn't be doing outreach for the Vasculitis Foundation, I wouldn't be chasing this dream I have, and I wouldn't be inspired to share my story with you.

But who knows, maybe it was destined to happen with my genetic makeup, my amazing support network, and a dreamer mind that likes to shoot for the top. So maybe it would have just happened another day in another way. One thing I can say is that I'm incredibly grateful for it to have happened with two of my best friends in tow. After that run it was clear to me that once the dirt was removed, there were still a bunch of embers under there that were ready to start a raging fire again in the pit of my stomach.

As time passed, and life has moved on, that run has become more and more important. In the fall of 2015 the world lost one of the brightest lights it has ever known--Cameron Bean (a.k.a. Cameron CronCity Magnum Bean)--to a hit and run accident in Chattanooga, Tennessee while out on a run. I feel the need to explain why he gets the long introduction each time. See Cameron was unapologetic about who he was. He went by the nicknames CronCity and Magnum, which he gave himself. When I was racing at Appalachian State he ran for another team in our conference, Samford University, and we absolutely hated him. When he moved to the mountains to train with Zap in 2010, he and I immediately became friends. Joining Zap was a leap for him. He hadn't run quite fast enough to meet any of the team's standards to garner support, but Pete Rea the coach had promised to coach Cameron (a.k.a. Cameron CronCity Magnum Bean) if he moved to the area. In the 16 year history of Zap Fitness Pete has made this promise to countless athletes, none have ever taken him up on the offer besides Cameron (a.k.a. Cameron CronCity Magnum Bean). He was sort of an outsider when he first arrived, not turning down any of his loud personality. Once he was on my side of the fence he became a true genuine friend. He helped me so much in the early stages of my semi-professional running career, and was of course there that fateful day when my life path changed in 2013. At times I felt like he was a bigger fan of me than I was of myself. That's Cameron and why he touched so many people's lives in his 28 short years on this flying rock.

The other half of that duo, Chris Moen, was a college teammate of mine at Appalachian who has since become a brother from another mother. We couldn't be more polarizing opposites as humans. I'm a high strung, high energy person and Moen is like a rock. He was a big proponent of me writing this book and so many of the ideas of this book have been hashed out with him on runs or while we were sitting around doing nothing. I can't tell you how many hours that we have spent discussing life and all the craziness that it brings. He and I have the ability to free think together. We can bounce ideas off each other as they come to our tongue without having to formulate the idea first. We do a lot of chewing on ideas together. He is a big part of the man that I have become today. He has helped me solidify my own views and personality through the sheer ability to be able to explore topics and ideas without judgment. That's why I picked him to do the foreword of this book.

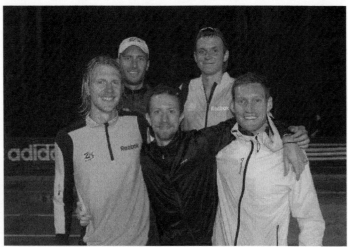

Front Row from left (Chris Moen, me, Cameron Bean aka CronCity Magnum Bean) Back Row from left (Ryan Warrenburg, Joe Stilin) (photo by Tim Meigs)

As it so often happens with friends, we now live in separate cities and our talks have to be crammed into phone calls and text messages. But every time we do talk, you can tell we both miss the ability to just sit and spend hours doing nothing but talking. In the two years that we lived together we never had cable television. We didn't need it.

Something big also happened in my life that year that I never saw coming. I was stopped in my tracks by a girl I had met the previous summer at a running camp, Ryanna. As of July that year we had been hanging out for a year without any real idea about what exactly our relationship was. In May of 2013 Ryanna did something I never saw coming.

She took two major steps during this time that I, quite frankly, would have never been able to make myself. The first was when, without any invocation, she decided to join me and sit with me during my fourth and final round of chemotherapy. Now, as anybody who has experienced or seen this process knows, it's not easy. Mine was made even worse by the fact that my doctor at the time was in Charleston, SC, a three-hour drive away from my home in Rock Hill. Ryanna, having only briefly met my parents, jumped in a car at 6:00 a.m., rode to Charleston with me, spent six hours with me while I got my infusion, and then sat through the three-hour ride home. Obviously a fun filled "first date" of sorts.

During these trips there wasn't a lot of talking. Your body is tired from taking in all the sludge you have just received via IV and your mind is just kind of lost in the pain and nausea. I, by no means, had anything close to a bad case. It's just what your body goes through, no matter how well your body can handle the abuse. At this point we had placed no label on what we were, nor had ever expressed interest in being more than we were. We simply got along and enjoyed each other's company.

While we were both quick to come to our defenses when people would ask about our relationship, it was clear to outsiders and friends that there was a lot more to it than we were letting on. Not only did she spend that chemotherapy day with me, but she spent a few days with me afterward as I kind of licked my wounds and started to attempt to get back to a life. It was a lot of lying around watching TV and doing nothing at all actually.

But what mattered was that she was there and I wasn't alone, and that meant the world to me. And, as if all this wasn't enough, she dropped the L bomb on me during that time and I, for the first time in years, was brought to tears. At one of my lowest points in life, here was someone with whom I had been sharing time during the last few years, which was a very dark and tumultuous time, and she somehow found something in me that she loved.

This was something that I knew myself, but something that I didn't know was reciprocated. I didn't have the strength at the time to be the one to say it. And if I had been the one it might have honestly come off as clingy and needy. My only regret with this was I hadn't been strong enough to say it before then. For her, it was a huge investment and step to take. For me I was just being pathetic and whiny and should've manned up and said it. That's not how it happened though. If she hadn't said it, then I don't know how long it would've gone on before I could've found the balls to be the one to bring that topic up.

Since then, Ryanna and I have been with each other through many more trials and tribulations. I wish I could say that it's been an easy four years since then, but with the lives we both lead, and our headstrong personalities, it's been up and down at times. No matter what we still love each other and are both willing to work (mainly on me not being a selfish asshole) to make each other happy and supported. She has been the only thing that could drag me off the mountain. Right before this book came out I finally took the plunge and moved in with her in Jamestown, North Carolina where she has been living the last 3 years. It finally got to be too much being away from each other.

At the risk of sounding cheesy, it couldn't have happened any other way. If I had been too pushy or she had been too pushy early in our relationship, then one of us would have scared the other away. We were both searching for something—but not a relationship. What we wanted was fun with no strings attached. It took a full two years of being around each other and sharing ourselves before we were ready for a commitment, and probably another year before we began openly referring to each other as boyfriend and girlfriend.

While I was in Graduate school at Appalachian State, a guy by the name of James Snyder joined the coaching staff as a Graduate Assistant coach. He was a smooth talking, shit-talker, and southerner at heart, from the outskirts of Philadelphia, PA. Just like anyone that has ever crossed paths with James, I was instantly a captive to his spell. Something about him, even though he is a year younger than me, made me buy into his philosophies. He also ain't afraid to talk a little shit, and then back it up. He was still in really good shape from his college racing days, and not long after he joined the squad as a coach in Boone he hopped in with us during the Firetower climb. It's been a staple of Appalachian State cross-country for over 20 years. The run is 5 mile hard climb up a set of carriage trails in Moses Cone Park where we often train. It's a workout done at the beginning of every cross-country season, when everyone has reported back from summer break. The atmosphere is always electric. People are excited to show off the hard work they have put in over the summer. It's serious enough that we keep an official team record. I had already notched two conference titles the year before on the track and put in a fantastic summer of training in Boone. James managed to leave me and many of my other teammates in the dust. About 4 miles up James even had time to stop, take a quick shit on the side of the trail, hop back out, and beat me by over a minute to the top. To this day he won't let me forget it.

I moved in with James shortly after finishing up my last season at Appalachian. We never sat down and had a discussion about it, but both just assumed that he was going to be my coach. We had nearly identical thoughts about training and both had big goals in the sport. Six years later, while we no longer have the benefit of living together or even being in the same city, he is still my coach and the only person I trust with my training. Sometimes I will want to fight him on something, but in the end he is always right. He knows the right buttons to press. It's the sign of a great coach. When I want to do too much, he reigns me in. When I'm being stupid and not checking off all the little things, James is in my grill reminding me to stay focused. Above all else he is a good listener. When things aren't going right or I have another feeling about something, James takes the time to listen and hear me out. For him, coaching me is just a side gig. He is now the Head Cross-Country and Assistant Track Coach at Temple University. Once he got a big program job, I wouldn't have faulted him for not taking the time to coach me. His kids at Temple are his number one priority. Luckily for me he hasn't told me to take a hike. He's been with me through hell and back over the past six years. I still want to make him proud. We have unfinished business on the track.

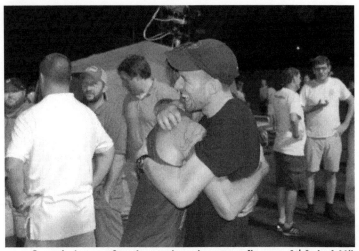

**Coach James Snyder embracing me after my 1ˢᵗ Sub 4 Mile
(photo by Calvin Hudgins)**

My poor parents. Emily and Calvin Hudgins have
had to endure things that no parent is ever
prepared for. When I was four years old, they lost
my baby sister, Allison Grace Hudgins, who was born
with a heart defect and only lived 19 days. Then, 16
years later, they had to watch as their oldest son
was diagnosed with some weird faceless disease. I
can't imagine the agony they went through during
those times. They are our family's rocks. And as I
look back on the really dark and depressing times I
experienced during those years, the thought of my
mom losing another child is what really kept me
alive.

Even though I was just four years old at the time of
Allison's death, I saw what it did to my family. When
those dark times occasionally come now, that

picture is even more clear to me at 30 than it was 20 or 24. My parents are the most loving people in the entire world and have really helped raise a community of kids in their time. The world is a better place because of them. I know that no matter what I choose in life they will always support and love me.

That is such a large part of who I have grown up to be. They have supported every crazy decision I've made even when they couldn't help me financially. They have always supported my efforts no matter how long the odds. It's the most lucky part of my life, being born to Calvin and Emily. Now, I just want to make them even more proud, take them with me when I travel and show them the world that they opened their son up to 30 years ago.

Last but certainly not least are my younger brother and sister, Tyler and Calli. I'm big brother and I know I've made life difficult for the two of them. Our family is insanely tough on each other for some reason. It's no-holds-barred when one of us screws up. As tough as it may be at times, it keeps each of us honest. Nobody in the world is quicker to call my bullshit than Tyler and Calli. Both have seen far too much from me over the years to accept one ounce of it from me. Growing up the three of us were never some lovey-dovey threesome that skipped and frolicked together. In fact, at times we made life a living hell. While I may have been tough on them at times, my only wish for each of them in life has always been for them to find their own way. Both chose to run cross-country and track, each being talented in their own rights, but have ultimately moved on to their own passions in life. We all share the same background in life, but have grown into three crazy adults now!

All of these people have made my journey a life worth living. Everyone that I've talked about, except Cameron (who had to join me in spirit), got to join me in Eugene, Oregon in July of 2016 to watch as I competed on the second highest stage in the sport of track and field, the U.S.A. Olympic Trials. It was a whirlwind of 10 days with so many ups and downs, but it makes my heart warm to have had all of them there. They were all the backbone of Team Brandon as I experienced ups and downs on my journey to the Trials. I don't mince words when I say that I would drop anything that I'm ever doing if any of them ever needs my help. Life for Vasculitis patients can be a major struggle and I'm incredibly lucky to have the support network that I have.

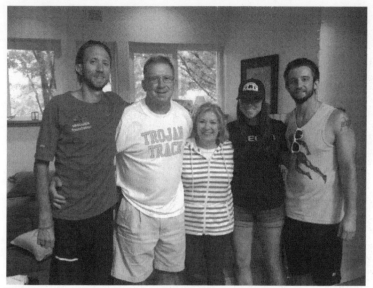

The Family at the Olympic Trials From left (Me, Dad, Mom, Calli, Tyler)

I share all of these stories about my support network because these people and others (whose stories I'd love to share) that make up my support network have been vital to my success. As much satisfaction as I get from doing things my way, it's this support network that allows that luxury. Without them I am nothing. When you go through challenging times in your life you will learn who really is there for your support.

Often these times will burn you to your core or plow a rut through your brain. It's going to hurt and probably get worse before it gets any better. It's one of the worst parts of experiencing tragic events in life. You expect the struggle from the event, but what often isn't talked about is the bailing of people you thought were important in your life.

One of the most common things I hear from discussions with patients in the vasculitis community is the loss of friends and loved ones. It's disheartening to hear stories of divorces and breakups during such trying times. I had my own experience with it at 20 when my girlfriend was cheating on me and then broke up with me the night before I was supposed to have surgery in March of 2008. It was late in the six month period of sickness that precluded my diagnosis with Vasculitis and those months were the most physically challenging of my life. While I can now say it was for the better (there were many reasons the relationship shouldn't have lasted, but the main one is that it was a teenage relationship that had outlasted its time), I can't imagine a spouse leaving me. I also became incredibly difficult to deal with as a teammate and roommate while I was finishing my time at Winthrop. 20 year olds aren't equipped with the skills to navigate the waters of a life threatening disease. I made being my friend tough, but many of my friends at the time also didn't step up to truly understand what I was going through. Now I harbor no ill will towards any of them, it's just unfortunately the nature of dealing with a rare life threatening illness while also trying to be a "normal" college student.

I've always maintained that you have to be ok with being alone before you can be with someone else. I have come to that conclusion because I fought much of those early days of my disease alone, and that gave me a lot of strength and taught me a lot about myself. So when I was ready to be in a relationship again, I had a strong understanding of who I was and what I wanted in life. I wasn't compromising with another person for my beliefs and goals.

When Ryanna and I both got together, there was an understanding that we both had goals and we would be supporting each other in our own journeys together. It's depressing at times when you realize how many relationships and friendships you lose when tragedy strikes, but it also solidifies and strengthens the ones you have. So don't cry over spilled milk, as the saying goes. Cherish the relationships you do have.

Also, realize that once you have been supported by these people, you may be called on to return the favor. True friendship has a nonzero sum. Be conscious of this. Don't be the one who is always asking for a favor, but never able to return it. I'm not saying you have to keep score. That's not the goal. But if one party begins to feel like he or she is the one who is constantly helping but not receiving, it can turn them off and drive them away. When you have true friendship, you want to be there for that person no matter what. Make sure that person feels the same love you feel from him or her.

Find your goal

How have I managed to find my way back to chasing my childhood dreams? It's plain and simple now. I know my goals. Whether they are written out for me or something I daydream about while I'm out running. I know what I want, I know what's required, and I do what's necessary. In order to succeed you have to find your goal and your why. You may lose focus on that goal occasionally, but if you have the right goal you will find your way back to it. When you commit, though, you have to be willing to do whatever it takes to make progress toward, and, eventually achieve your goal.

It can't be half-assed. If it is, you won't make it during the tough times. Find friends and family members who will help you by holding you accountable. And—ultimately—keep yourself accountable.

During the early days of my first comeback after my initial battle with Vasculitis, I would write my goals down on Post-it notes or slips of paper and stick them on my bathroom mirror or the back of my bedroom door. They served as constant reminders to myself that I value this journey. Once you have committed fully to the journey, though, you don't need little sticky notes and cheesy reminders of why you are chasing this dream. You start to live it.

The feeling becomes contagious and addicting, so you will do what is necessary to keep that feeling.

There really is no artificial high that can mimic the everyday euphoria of living your dream! Believe me. I've chased highs and rushes in all sorts of ways when I lost sight of my goals. Some of them will even get the job done temporarily, but there is always the next morning, if you get my drift.

You have to constantly challenge yourself to grow along the journey. Doing that will ensure that you stay on the right path and follow your steps to your goals. Here is a brief look at what my goal and steps were like during my third comeback that lead to a sub-four-minute mile and then the Olympic Trials in 2016:

Goal: break four-minute mile

Steps:
1. GPA remission
2. Start running again
3. Start racing again
4. Break four-minute mile
5. Qualify for the Olympic Trials

These goals were simple and easy for me to follow in my head. After my second relapse and a bout with anxiety and depression in 2014 I had a new outlook and I no longer needed the sticky notes to remind me what I wanted. Upon reflection the steps were much more complex and looked more like this:

1. Put GPA/Wegener's into remission
2. Start running again

3. Find a job that allows me the flexibility to train and race while making enough money
4. Start training with a purpose
5. Gain the confidence to race again
6. Run personal best at longer distances
7. Find the love for racing again
8. Get fit enough to compete
9. Find the zone and get it done on race day
10. Finally break 4 minutes in the mile
11. Get a sponsorship
12. Run a Qualifying time for the 2016 Olympic Trials

When I first decided to focus on breaking the four-minute mile I had no idea what it would take to get from step one to step four—much less all the other steps I would have to go through to get there. But as new challenges arose, I augmented my plan without losing sight of the goal. This process took more than two years from the time I began running again to being in the position to break four minutes. Then, it took an additional year to prepare to run even faster to qualify for the Olympic Trials. Once these goals were achieved I was ready to move on to the next set of goals—which was to live my dream: having a career as a professional distance runner. See, I couldn't live the professional lifestyle until I did certain things. Much like you can't become a doctor without first graduating from college and medical school, serving a residency and passing the boards. It takes a plan, time, tenacity, and making modifications when needed.

So, make a plan and be both dedicated and flexible.

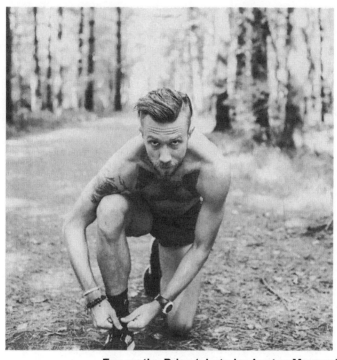

Eye on the Prize (photo by Austen Mauney)

Find Your Why

You can't understand your goals if you don't understand your why. The why can be as simple as, you just want to, or as complex as because you want to save the world one child at a time. People start chasing a dream for a million different reasons. You see from my story that the "why" can even change from time to time. It's important to know your why so you can accurately know how. If you read nothing else from this book, read this:

Without a why, what does anything you do mean?

Finding the why in your journey may take some serious self-exploration, but it is the key to this entire book. Desire breeds dedication. Desire comes through your why. You cannot take the first step on your journey towards your dream without figuring out your desires and ambitions. Not having a desire or ambition is one thing that I think causes people to become complacent and stagnant, and therefore unhappy in life. If you don't have a why to live for, then is life really worth living? Because of the pressures of our society and many others like it, people often find themselves in a rut doing a job that they hate or in which they find no pleasure.

They may have had a dream at one point in high school or college, but that dream took a backseat to bills, a career, societal pressures, and other things. Maybe that dream seemed far-fetched and unattainable, or was discouraged by family members or loved ones. Whatever the reason, many Americans have lost sight of their dreams and passions for a more mundane life that offers safety and security. I'm not saying that there aren't people who find happiness in security. Maybe you're one of them, and that is your why.

But for those who have security and still feel unsatisfied, I truly believe they might be doing the wrong things in life. If you take the first step to figuring out what your desires are, then just maybe you will find the ambition to chase your dream. Once you find your why, it's important to realize that you may fail, but going for it will ultimately bring you happiness.

As you grow older, you often lose track of memories and emotions. I still remember begging my Dad to let me run my first race at age 10 in the fall of 1997. Our neighbor, Coach Tice, was the local club coach and also my dad's assistant track and cross-country coach. I grew up playing soccer with Tice's son, and Tice had been asking me for a while to join the cross-country club. It just so happened that his club was hosting the Youth USATF State Cross-Country meet that year and I decided that I really wanted to be involved. At this time, I hadn't been to a practice, nor had I run further than probably a mile in my entire life. At the time my bedroom walls were covered with posters of Joe Montana, Dwight Clark, Jerry Rice, Steve Young, Larry Johnson, Michael Jordan, and other sports heroes; my sports heroes. Note that there wasn't a runner among them. No, I was dreaming of being the next big-time NFL quarterback or playing point guard in the NBA.

But for some reason I really wanted to run. Nineteen years is a long time to think back on, so I can't seem to remember exactly why I was so passionate about wanting to run. Maybe it was because it was different than what I'd been doing or maybe it was because my friend was doing it. Maybe I didn't even really know why. Dad didn't believe that I should be going out to run a race and do a sport I had never practiced. He believed that positions needed to be earned. Still, my enthusiasm didn't wane in the weeks leading up to the race. I begged my parents to let me do it, despite them repeatedly giving me a big fat NO every time. Finally—and thankfully—they caved when they realized it was something that I was willing to fight for.

But Dad still wasn't convinced that I could even run the three-kilometer race distance (just short of 2 miles). So, during the week leading up to the race, he took me to the site of the race, Winthrop University Farm, and told me that if I could complete the one-mile loop around the lake there twice without stopping that I could do the race. Well, much to his dismay, I made it all the way around— not once, but twice. So he held up his end of the bargain and allowed me to race.

Come race day that October on a chilly Saturday morning, I set off with a bunch of other skinny, awkward 10-year-olds to race three kilometers. With this being my first race and it being fairly cold outside, my mom over dressed me in sweats, hats, gloves, and layers to keep me from freezing to death. Well, by the time I had passed my competitors on the first loop of the course, I had shed more than half my clothes and was carrying them in my hands. In my first race I placed in the top 10 and helped our team qualify for the regional race two weeks later in Asheville, NC. The running bug had bit me and I have never looked back.

I often wonder at times just what it was about the sport that grabbed my attention at such a young age and never let go. I often think about the hours that I spent at high school track practice with my dad and playing backyard football, drawing up plays to win the Super Bowl for the San Francisco 49ers, my favorite team. Something made me choose running over football and the reasons for that decision are lost on 30-year-old me. In the 19 years since I started running, I have run for many different reasons, quit for different reasons, and fallen in love with the sport so many different times.

My teenage self definitely ran as a way to fit into a group. Being so skinny (like most runners) and different from many others in my age group, I was often picked on as a middle school and high school student because of my size. Being good at running gave me a sense of purpose and an identity when I struggled to find that as an awkward teenager. It wasn't a classic identity, but it did fit right in with my outlaw rock- and-roll look anyway.

During my senior year of high school and my first two years at Winthrop University, I definitely ran to prove to people that I could be one of the best in the state and in the country. I felt overlooked by some of the bigger schools that I thought should be recruiting me, so I was on a mission to prove all of them wrong. This fed into my rebellious nature and helped stoke the fire to train hard and race even harder.

This fire, though, would come under attack during my junior and senior year of college when I was diagnosed with Vasculitis. As I've said, the disease took me away from competing for two years. After six months of being deathly sick and an additional six months of undergoing chemotherapy and taking hardcore (prescription) drugs, my body was wiped out, but my mind was ready to get back to running. I was convinced that I was going to beat the disease, put it in the rearview mirror and move on with my competitive running career.

That happened, but not easily, and I was given the opportunity to finish my two years of college eligibility at Appalachian State University while getting my Master's degree in exercise science. I quickly adapted to the "mountaineer lifestyle." The team's work ethic was infectious and in my first year helped my school win indoor and outdoor Southern Conference team titles, notching two individual crowns, one at 800 meters and the other at 1500 meters, along the way. My fire to train and compete with my teammates was back and as strong as ever. At this point I wasn't running as much for myself as I was for my team. I drew tremendous pride from putting on the block "A" uniform and competing beside my teammates. The team had welcomed me with open arms when I was still on the shelf, so to speak, and their attitudes helped elevate my mood and make me excited to train again. We were a ragtag cast of characters who took a lot of pride in training hard and playing hard. This was the sense of belonging I had been searching for since I was in middle school. We had a Yoda like coach, I had my ragtag group of friends who believed in me, and I believed in them. When a team has the same goal and a like-mindedness, special things can happen.

I often look back at some of the races my teammates and I ran on tired legs. I look at it with a sense of wonder (because I couldn't fathom doing it now), but in the moment all the pain was as smooth as a hot knife through butter. When you are in the zone, the pain is clean and the stakes are high, but it seems effortless in retrospect. There were days and times when you felt like you could run through a brick wall if the team needed your points. But these moments don't last forever. We all grow out of team sports, or our current situations. The trick is taking the next steps to make sure that your why is still meaningful.

Now I put on my singlet with the Vasculitis Foundation logo and feel the hundreds and even thousands of people behind me who have been impacted by my story. My why has changed since college but it wasn't an easy transition without several failures. The transition from team running to being a professional with purely selfish desires, was one that was tough to navigate. It was easy to quit on myself at times; I had a lot of lonely runs and workouts with no one looking when it was easy to just walk away once it became super tough. There are times when I'm out at the track or on the trails and the workout is getting tough and I'll start finding excuses to stop instead of finding the reasons to forge on.

I'd be lying if I said I'd made the transition smoothly. It didn't help that I'd suffered two relapses from my GPA during these two years—but, regardless, I think I would have found moments when it was just hard for me to continue. Each time, I would fight back with a vengeance the first few months. But inevitably, as things started to plateau and the progress slowed, I would find it hard at times to stay focused and get myself over the edge.

The saying that champions are born when no one is watching this is true. The little moments, the little battles - although failures in the short term, were lessons in the long run. I got so accustomed to getting up from the mat and starting to swing again that once I was on my feet and I wasn't immediately knocked back down, I was kind of groundless. I would create my own problems, find things to stress about and make mountains out of molehills, as the saying goes.

As we grow and learn, often the why will change for everyone. The trick is in making sure to continue to ask why, and be comfortable not knowing at times. Life happens, and circumstances and people change. I may still be running to prove people wrong and feel like I belong, but that's not the only reason now. As I said previously, anger and bitterness can't sustain me anymore. For a lot of people, getting married, having kids, experiencing the death of loved ones, and other significant events changes them. Those things have a way of plowing a rut through your brain that changes your goals and mission in life.

While I may not have kids, I've seen so many of my peers and friends have them. It changes you and changes why you do things. If we remain the same selfish person through these types of events, then we aren't growing and learning. There's a saying, "We get old, we stop learning." Make sure you take time from year to year or even from event to event to remind yourself why you are doing something. You might find out that what you have been chasing is no longer what you want in life. That's fine too, but you have to be honest with yourself.

As you have seen, my why has changed a lot in just the last 15 years of my short life. When you have your why, that means your life has a goal or a meaning. The small things that then pop up become a lot less important and a lot less stress.

Prepare for Failure

Just because I had a wonderful plan didn't mean that I wouldn't fail a lot along the way or have to make extreme adjustments. Learning to be flexible and roll with the punches is the key to keeping your eyes on the prize. You can't be so rigid that you don't have room for failure or falls. Virtually everyone experiences setbacks. Even though you have your goal and the necessary steps laid out, it doesn't mean you're going to have a direct path.

Plan for failure. Why? Because if you don't fail or fall along the way, quite frankly, you aren't trying hard enough. Being prepared to deal with setbacks is the strongest tool you have on your journey to find your center. My path might seem like it was all uphill from my last relapse in 2013 to the Olympic Trials in the summer of 2016, but that couldn't be farther from the truth. Looking back on it, I can see and feel the upward trajectory, but it doesn't take away those dark moments when the odds were stacked against me or I was suffering from a panic attack, missing runs because I had to work too late, missing races because I couldn't get off work, or losing confidence in my ability to race at a high level and, as a result, got my clock cleaned in a race..

Getting over the fear of failing and realizing that everything is going to be alright is what taking risk is all about. Often in distance running, a coach will ask an athlete to go out hard in a race and hit splits that the athlete thought might not be possible.

Sometimes you don't know what you can accomplish until you try. And sometimes, when the coach is asking an athlete to do this, it's because the athlete is fit and ready physically, but might not have the confidence to hold that pace yet. So by laying the aggressive splits out there for the athlete, the coach is forcing the athlete to confront that pace. Now, I've been on both sides of this situation as an athlete and coach. For some reason it's very scary as an athlete, because we all have nightmares about the big blowup. But to quote one of the top distance running coaches in the USA, Alberto Salazar, "Don't be afraid of the blowup. It's a learning lesson."

If you go out hard and hit the aggressive splits this time, you are that much more prepared for the next time. And next time usually works. Your body responds to the rigorous pace, and you aren't in foreign territory anymore. Now, I may be using the word risk, but risks are calculated based on lots of data from training and how the body has adapted. Taking a "risk" is only smart if you are prepared. It might look like a risk to outsiders, but in reality it's not a risk if you're prepared to handle it. It's your path to success and not really a risk at all. More on this later though.

Making a big decision in life to chase your goals may come with some risk, but you have to prepare for them. That's why laying out goals and checkpoints along the way are important. Then, when it's time to take that leap, you're prepared and aren't leaping blindly off a cliff. It's like jumping off a high dive at your local pool; you know the pool is deep enough, but there is still a risk that you could land on your back and knock your wind out. If you practice enough and spend enough time doing it, the risk for failure becomes very low. Not preparing for your leap? Well, that's like jumping off a bridge into a river and you don't know how deep the water is. You may still succeed, but the risks are far greater for failure. No matter how much experience you have jumping off high dives or cliffs, you wouldn't want to jump into a river that may appear to be deep enough, but might not be relative to the risk you're taking. So set up your steps and practice, and be prepared. Then, leap with assertiveness.

Now when you take your leap, one of two things will happen: you will nail it, or you will fall flat on your face and have to pick yourself up. If you nail it, things are simple. You take the positives and you move on to your next step or challenge. If you fail, though, things can get murky. These are moments from which to learn. So you failed. So what? It feels super-depressing when you do. If you let yourself though, you can slide all the way back to step one.

But that's not why you're reading this book. You're reading it because you want to get better and make changes and learn from your mistakes. You've already taken the most difficult step—getting started—so don't stop just because you failed. If you stop, you'll have to summon the courage to start all over again. Think about all the people who join gyms at the beginning of each year as part of a New Year's resolution. After a few weeks they inevitably quit. It gets hard; they miss a few workouts and things get in the way. They are destined for failure because they didn't plan for success.

So what you missed a workout? Or maybe you bombed a job interview for your dream position? You quit your old job and now you are going to run out of money. You thought you nailed it. It wasn't part of the plan to not get it. That's why I generally live by the 48-hour rule. I allow myself to be upset, mad, sad, angry, stressed for 48 hours. After that, if I don't work on getting out of that funk it can become unhealthy. It's necessary that you get that emotion out, because when those 48 hours are over, you better be ready to get back to work.

How do we do this? We go back to our goals and steps. Where did we mess up? Was it just execution? Was it poor planning? Was it the wrong mindset? When you fail you have to take a hard look at yourself and be honest. Take ownership in that failure. If you don't, you are deflecting and you won't be ready for the next leap. Admit you screwed up. It's okay. I've failed more times than I can count at relationships, friendships, job interviews, decision-making, and workouts. I've also failed in races on the biggest stages. What I've learned through all of this, and what I want to share with you is that it's okay to fail. It's okay to work really hard for something and not get it. But if you are ever going to be satisfied with the journey, you have to be honest in your assessment of your failures. That's where you learn and grow. If you stop learning and growing, you might as well stop and give up now. So if you have to, look at yourself in the mirror and tell yourself you failed. You will be stronger for it.

To use my steps above as an example, consider this:

In 2014, a year before I broke four minutes in the mile, I came agonizingly close with a 4:01 clocking and several 1500-meter races (the metric mile) that were right at the four-minute mile conversion. I had spent so many years on that side of the barrier and been in sub-four-minute shape several times, but could just never catch the right break. So I was frustrated. Then, because of my work schedule, I missed a few races for chances to qualify for the USA Nationals and I was ready to quit. At 27 it seemed like there were just too many obstacles preventing me from making the jump to the next level. I felt like I had to get the stars to align to be in the right situation. Add to that my lack of big-time performances over the past few years and it was getting tougher and tougher to get into races. So from May that year (when I ran 4:01) until July, I was just going through the motions. I had let the journey get away from me and the mountain seemed insurmountable again.

In the running world we live and die by our times. Those silly numbers on the clock often dictate who we are as a person. They are how we got a college scholarship, how we get into certain races, and our ability to make money as professionals. There are two terms that are often used when it comes to these times: personal best (PB) and personal record (PR). These terms, which are often used interchangeably, refer to our best times over a given distance. So for instance my PR for the mile is 3:59.67 and my PR for 1500 meters is 3:38.20. I know these and so many other of my PR's by heart. The track and field world uses the PR and PB words interchangeably, but in reality they can be vastly different marks.

Today, I consider PBs and PRs to be two completely different things. I have learned time and time again that often your best on a given day might not be a record for you. Sometimes the circumstances dictate what your best will be, and that may not always be your personal record, or PR. For a long time during my 20s, through comeback after comeback, my PBs and PRs were vastly different. On the day in 2008 when I ran a mile non-stop for the first time since being diagnosed with GPA, my PB that day was well over 10 minutes, which was technically over 6 minutes slower than my PR. Of course, that was a long way from the 4:06 mile PR that I owned at the time, but on that day, I gave every ounce of energy in my body to complete that task. So it had to be a PB. Your PB is often fluid. Just weeks before my first nonstop mile in 2008, my PB was based on running for a minute without stopping. Before that it was based on getting out of the house and going for a walk. I had an incredible desire to get back to the level of athlete I had been, but it didn't happen overnight. It came through small victories in my PB each and every week along the way.

As I've said before, I've been lucky enough to be in remission from my Vasculitis for long enough periods during which I have been able to chase PR's again and not just PB's. Not all Vasculitis patients are that lucky. I know that there are thousands of Vasculitis patients and others suffering from debilitating diseases that may never be in good enough health to accomplish similar physical feats. That's why always striving for a PB each day is so important, regardless of your lot in life.

The important part of learning to fight like hell is defining what a PB and PR are going to mean for you. That's why it's so critical to set goals. My goal was to get back on my journey to becoming a professional distance runner. For others, the goal might just be to walk around the block without stopping, finish a degree that had to be postponed, figure out how to change careers mid-life, get out of debt, learn to play an instrument, or any of the other millions of possible goals in life. There are always going to be obstacles and things that can hold people back from achieving their goals. The commitment you have to make is with yourself, and that is to consistently achieve your PB. If you consistently strive for a PB on your journey, you will soon find yourself redefining your PB and those steps towards your ultimate goal will look a lot easier to accomplish.

The mountain of any goal can be daunting. That's why having your steps laid out and reaching for a PB instead of big PRs is so important to the process. Continually looking for PRs isn't sustainable. When you're a kid, things often come to you easily. I remember back in high school when I got better at sports not always by working harder or smarter, but just simply by being alive longer. The process generally continues in college, as maturation plays a huge part in success. As we age and adult life begins to happen, the big jumps in performance we enjoyed early on in our careers become much harder to achieve. This situation can become frustrating, and is often the downfall of many high-level athletes. I've been a victim of it myself at times. Now that's not to say that hard work didn't play a part in my success in high school, college, and professionally, but hard work was aided by a still maturing body. Now that I'm 30 the gains come in much smaller increments, but need to be celebrated just like the big ones. From ages 13 to 20 I went from a PR in the mile of 4:50 down to 4:06. It then took another seven years to get from 4:06 to 3:59.

Chasing any dream isn't much different. Let's apply it to when an alcoholic or addict decides to become sober. The big initial step, before actually getting clean, is making the decision to get clean. For a person who has been an addict for years, the first week is huge. The first month is huge. Then, six months is huge, then one year, then two years, and so on. Those first few milestones of one week and one month aren't any less important than a week at the eight-year mark. A week sober is a week sober, and that should be celebrated. The people experiencing this have also redefined their personal best and personal records, so a week is no longer as big of a deal as it initially was.

Those first few weeks and months, while they were difficult and challenging, came quickly. It's fighting those same urges after years of battles and trying to return to a normal life that a lot of people find challenging. That's why it's always going to be work staying sober and fighting that demon. Every week above ground sober should be celebrated for the addict, but if he or she never moved beyond these small battles, they would never make it back into a normal life. But if they let their guard down and slip it starts the process all over again. Just as fighting for a PR later in life can take a long time, that doesn't make it any more or less important than the check marks along the way.

All PBs and PRs involve a realignment of personal standards. To constantly grow in life, we have to examine where we are at on our journey.

Routines

Routine, routine, routine, routine. I can't say that word enough. Successfully changing any bad habits requires a modification in your routine. If you are going to make any significant change in your lifestyle, your emotional state or elsewhere, you will have to change your approach and your routine.

A lot can be learned from observing successful business people or athletes. Anytime you read one of those click-bait articles like "Five Things All Success People Do," you will see routine mentioned somewhere on that list, every time, guaranteed. Why is that? Well I can tell you from experience that when you set a routine, it requires less mental energy to accomplish a task. When you are in a good routine, tasks take care of themselves.

Now, at this point, I could dig into the science behind circadian rhythms and hormone levels, and how they affect productivity. But what it all really boils down to is the fact that our bodies crave patterns and routines. They allow our body to know what's coming so it can be prepared to deal with the tasks at hand. We all have our own quirks that make up our daily routine, but no matter how weird that routine is, it's important to stick to one. It creates structure for your day and allows you to be more productive with your time.

One reason many successful people have such a good work ethic is because they compartmentalize those moments in time when they need to work. Obviously, this can be taken to an extreme. But generally speaking, if you set aside time to accomplish the tasks that you need to do, you will be less likely to get less distracted and become more productive. Today, with the Internet and social media at our fingertips 24/7, it's easy to get distracted, and, before you know it, you've lost 30 minutes to meaningless scrolling.

When I was a professional athlete, I often had to follow a strict routine in order to balance training time and a full-time job, and I had little time for distractions. This made for some extremely productive moments, but it also led to extreme amounts of stress at times because of the lack of time (which we cover in the section on bad stress). On the other hand, it's how I managed to get my ass out the door at 10:00 or 11:00 p.m. for a second run three or four days a week.

I had my routine, knew what needed to be done and didn't have time to waste, because if I did that I would lose time for sleeping, which would affect my recovery, mood and the next day's training. When you have your why figured out and have the desire to accomplish a goal, it's important to find a routine to help you get there as effectively as possible. It might require investing in long hours and experiencing some tough times, but once you get there it will be incredibly gratifying.

So how do we break from old habits and form new habits and routines for your goals? Think of breaking a habit or routine as forming a new one. Research has determined that the time it takes to form new habits varies from person to person, so it could happen in as few as 18 days or as long as 200-plus days. This is why you shouldn't become discouraged if you're still finding it difficult to break an old habit and form a new one after a month.

Many people make resolutions or commitments, but often struggle to stick it out for the time it takes to form a new routine. They come for a few days the first week, two or three days the second and maybe one day the third. Then, they just stop going at all. They haven't spent the time it takes to make a new routine to replace an old one. The same can be said for chasing your dream by following the steps to your goal. If you find yourself constantly starting and stopping you will never stay committed long enough to form new habits. I will say that this is where the discipline of being a distance runner has paid off and transformed other parts of my life.

Like most athletes, we distance runners live and die by our routines. We practice and eat meals at the same times every day. We have pre-race and pre-workout rituals that have to be done to ensure optimal performance in both practice and competition. This pattern of behavior helped me write this book and do many other things in my career under a time constraint. With runs and weight routines that needed to be done each day, plus eating, naps and, of course, working to make a living, the window of time I had for writing was very narrow and I needed to be productive while I was in front of my computer. So on each day I planned to write I made sure to set aside the time, put my phone on silent and promise myself to stay off Facebook and YouTube. It wasn't always easy, but once I got in a routine of coming home each day from my workouts and eating, I then had a narrow window in which to write, so I had to make it count. Some of my most productive thoughts and chapters from this book came during these early afternoon sessions where I only had an hour to write and I wanted to get as much as I could out and on paper.

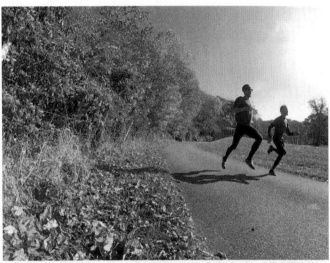

Training with my friend Andy Hash (photo by Bill Wilde)

How to Be Productive

So how can we go from being lazy, tired, worn-out, angry, bitter, depressed, and just ready to give up to insanely productive? Where does the switch or the willpower come from to make the necessary changes in our routines to produce the results? How do we get focused enough to conquer the huge life changes or goals we so desire?

Well the key is desire. I know I mentioned it earlier, but this is where it becomes important--desire breeds dedication. If you want something badly enough you'll find a way to have it. Now of course, you will also have hiccups and falls. It won't be a smooth ride and it may take several attempts at changing your habits. Lord knows I've failed more times than I'd like to admit, but you have to continually find ways to remind yourself of your goal. It's easy in the moment to give into the small things and not follow through on a routine or a promise you made to yourself. It's easy to go out with friends one night, stay out way too late, get shit sleep, and wake up and not be productive the next day. Sometimes it's even necessary. But when those little distractions break your routine and you can't get back to it, that's when they become a problem.

Find a way to continually remind yourself of your goals. Maybe you have to make sticky notes or big goal sheets and post them around your house or office. Maybe it means putting them above your bed, so they're the first and last things you see every morning.

When I returned to serious competitive racing after my second relapse with GPA, I wrote down my time goals for the season along with the question, "How are you getting closer today?" on a note card and taped it to the footboard of my bed. This was my daily reminder for the first year.

Today, I don't need it as I've since found my routine and inner motivation. But that year I needed that reminder each and every day. Oh, I still failed a number of times that first year, but I also ultimately found myself again. After that, I didn't have to wake up and go to sleep next to a note card with "sub 4" written on it in bright red marker. We have so many wonderful pieces of technology and apps that can help remind us of things we need to do now, there is no reason anyone should ever forget anything anymore. But we are still human, so of course we will find ways to get distracted (or go to the grocery store to get bananas, and accidentally leave with $100 worth of groceries you weren't intending to buy).

The other danger of being such a strong-minded person is that I can convince myself that almost anything is good for me. When you spend your life forcing yourself to be uncomfortable and pushing your limits, you also can teach yourself to justify things you know are bad. For example, one of my all time favorite comments to myself is, "You've earned this night out. You've been working hard.

You need a release. You've done it in the past and it's been fine. Go get obliterated with your friends, have fun and turn off for a night. You'll blow off some steam and be better for it."

Breaks are needed, but unhealthy habits and breaks aren't good. As someone who has studied the human body and its physiological responses, I know drinking myself into oblivion isn't good for my health, and especially isn't good for my decision-making skills. But time and time again I find myself convincing myself that I need it. It's important to identify these demons and thoughts and learn how to ignore them or divert our energy elsewhere. Because for all the times I've woken up with a hangover and been able to get back out the door and train and be fine, there have also been many times when I've gotten up sick. It's caused me to lose training time, get even sicker, go on antibiotics, and ultimately put myself behind the eight ball in an unnecessary way.

While I wish that writing this down and sharing it with you will help me curb this problem, I'll also admit that I'll probably fail again at some point. As it's been said, we all have our vices--so I just work to push those mistakes further and further apart from each other, until they are non-existent. Honestly, I could probably write an entire book on the mistakes I've made while out on the town (or even in my room alone) that have originated from this mindset. So be wary of this pattern.

Since realizing this pattern a few years ago, I have gotten much better about it. It was something that used to happen one or two times a month. I now have it down to just a few times a year and plan to eliminate it completely one step at a time. My routine helps me with this now. Fear of getting out of my routine has helped drive this number way down.

We all are at risk for taking backward steps when we are out of our routines. For me, that's when I'm on the road, traveling for races and taking breaks from training. That's why I also get so frustrated now during the holidays; they screw up my routines. I've become such a slave to my routines that I now run on Christmas morning before I even open presents, just to make sure that I have a good workout. If I didn't, I'd sit there opening presents while worrying about the run I needed to do later in the day.

It's so funny because as much as I love and crave a routine, I also love traveling for races and to see friends and family, which is a total cluster**** when it comes to getting in the work that needs to be done. Traveling to and from races goes smoothly about 95 percent of the time, but when you travel 20-plus weeks a year every year, then that means that something is going to go wrong. So you have to learn to be flexible, not get overly regimented and be a good problem solver if you are still going to arrive at your destination in time. As all travelers know, there are flights that are going to be canceled or delayed and you are going to get stuck somewhere. When you get stuck on a layover or are forced to land somewhere else due to weather, you sometimes have to be creative to get to the racing venue. Keeping a clear mind and a level head are key components of that process. Planes, trains and automobiles play crucial roles in the life of a traveling distance runner.

Well, those things and Google. I've seen many passengers throw temper tantrums over flight delays and cancellations due to things that are out of the airlines' control (on the other hand, a broken plane or bad management is different). One thing my years traveling on my own have taught me is how to keep calm when obstacles arise, and realize that there is (probably) still a way to get to my destination. If there is, I'll be able to find it. If not, well--I'm out of luck and will probably be sleeping in the airport. It won't be the first time I've done that and, as much as I dislike having to; it may not be the last either.

Racing for a living is stressful enough, and adding travel problems to the experience completely undoes some people. I've gotten in at 2 or 3 a.m. the night before a race and managed to put together a good race the next day, while I've seen others just completely bomb. They'll complain about the lack of sleep, not being able to get their normal pre-race meal or having to spend too much time in the airport. There's an old saying--shit happens. And when shit like that happens, you have two ways to react: roll with the punches, which is what I've learned to do, or get hit on the chin and knocked down.

Bend with the Wind

I've expressed the importance of having a consistent routine, and you know by now how much Importance I place on mine. But here's the deal: although a routine is very important to everyday life, you also can't become a slave to it. In my daily training, as well as in my life, I will sometimes do stuff the night before a big workout that is way out of my routine, just to make sure that I am not getting hung up on making sure everything is perfect. To quote my favorite martial artist and philosopher, Bruce Lee

"Notice that the stiffest tree is most easily cracked, while the bamboo or willow survives by bending with the wind."

Another thing that has helped me in this process is not being on a team. Distance running is a solo sport, and instead of having teammates I have a huge support network that includes coaches and trainers planning my every step for me. Sometimes I've shown up at tracks or gyms to run or lift and found myself locked out (oh, the joys of being a "professional" track athlete). Surprises like that force me out of my routine and I have to call an audible and figure out how to get the work done under the new circumstances. So if I find myself in the middle of Michigan and need to get to South Indiana in a snowstorm to an indoor track meet that's my last chance to qualify for the national meet, I learn not to freak out. Just like I want this book be a tool to chase your dream, I've acquired the tools to succeed in a variety of tough situations.

How do you get to the point where you can roll with the punches and not get your underpants in a wad? Well it's as simple as this:

One day at a time.
One mistake at a time.
One success at a time.

Success comes from the culmination of hours of hard work. If you let one day make or break your journey, then you will always fail. There were countless times on my journey that I had to switch workout days, skip runs, or miss a session simply because the stress of life had caught up to me. At the beginning of my journey, each one of these bumps used to burn me to my core. You need to be able to step back and see your journey as a whole and not focus on the minor details of one specific day. For instance, if you look at the training of a distance runner for a whole year or cycle, then you can understand how each day and workout adds up to the whole. Looking at the bigger picture you understand how taking out one or two pieces isn't catastrophic to the goal. On your journey through life you will experience challenges that will test your routine or plan. Don't let one of those derail the whole process.

It also helps to reward yourself for small victories along the way. All the hard work you put in toward a goal can and will be exhausting and frustrating.

Without rewards along the way, you won't make it. So treat yourself and set up rewards for certain goals obtained along your journey. What's success worth if you can't celebrate and enjoy your accomplishments?

Taking Risk

It might sound like I'm describing risk in the previous section and maybe to a certain extent I am but use of that word as it's applied to life absolutely aggravates me. I feel like it is so often used because many people don't understand the steps others have to take to achieve something out of the ordinary. If you've done your homework and are ready to be committed to seeing a goal through to the end, then it is by no means a risk. It's not dangerous; it's adventurous and freeing. What's risky is being stuck in a life or job that isn't fulfilling. That's what leads to dangerous behavior and thoughts. I know for me, personally, my darkest and most dangerous moments came when I was stuck in places that I hated: stuck with people I hated, stuck in a job I hated and had no direction in life. This was dangerous to both my mental and physical health. What's even worse, I didn't know how destructive these patterns were until I had pulled myself out of this cycle (with help from my real friends) and was able to see my goals clearly.

Now that you are empowered and ready to chase your dream, you have to take that big step. Let go of the things that are holding you back and take the leap. To many on the outside, this will look like a risk, but--again--I hate that word. Risk sounds like you aren't prepared. The word risk means there is an exposure to danger or harm. In our case, the danger or harm is failure. But when you are prepared, it's not a risk, it's your best chance for success.

If you embrace the challenge and dream as a risk, then you are giving into failure as an option. I have always felt that labeling something a risk is dis-empowering. The challenge should empower you, not be looked at as a threat. Doing so engages the wrong pathways in your brain. This is something you have to do to succeed, not something you are hoping (you know how I feel about that word) will work. Empower yourself by believing in your plan and your talents, and you will be able to take the necessary steps to succeed.

The "Risks" I've Taken

I've taken many big "risks" in my lifetime, but none bigger than quitting my day job as a guest services representative at a resort one month before the Olympic Trials in 2016. At the time I was working at the resort for nearly three years (my last day would be just a few days shy of the three-year mark). This job had provided me with a livable income, health insurance and a chance to live where I enjoy training. But the job, like many others I've held over the last six years, have come at a cost. Working and juggling the training and travel schedule of a professional track and field athlete is nearly impossible.

For those 3 years my daily schedule would often look like this:

8:30am - Wake Up

9:30am - Personal Training session
11:00am - my owning training (running, lifting weights, etc..)
1:30pm-2:00pm - cram food in my mouth
2:00pm-2:30pm - power nap
3:00pm - 11:00pm - guest services work
11:30pm - 2nd run
12:30am - bedtime

Doing this four to five days a week for several years will wear you thin. I had no time for myself, my relationship with my girlfriend or to devote to my passions or hobbies. It was all work, no play and very little enjoyment. Although I was able to grow and develop as a runner during this time period, I also developed a lot of problems. My anxiety was a constant battle, my depression would go through deep swings and my running became too stressful because I looked at it as my only escape from a job I didn't enjoy.

Eventually, my relationship with my girlfriend became a text message relationship, which isn't healthy. All these things began to pile up one after the other. In the beginning I had a lot of it under control, but little-by-little, more things in my life began to unravel. This was ironic because during this time I managed to have several big breakthroughs in my running career, but was at an all time low with some of my personal goals. I had been succeeding on the track, but failing in life with very little time to enjoy myself.

This burned me at my core. Part of who I am as a person means following a goal to its completion and successful outcome, but this was starting to become a nightmare for me. I wasn't having as much fun as I should have been. I had no time for myself. I had no time to grow as a person. And I wasn't able to give the time to my new work with the Vasculitis Foundation which was bringing me tremendous joy.

I knew deep down that I needed a change, but I was a slave to a paycheck and the stability that it provided. I needed money to chase my dream, since I had no shoe sponsorship to finance my running. I needed health insurance in case the unthinkable were to happen. And, I had to pay my bills, which running alone wasn't doing. So I felt stuck.

During this time I had some great accomplishments but also bombed beautifully. Every time I stood at the starting line of a race, I dreamed of that race being the one that would finally allow me the opportunity to be a full time athlete. But guess what? That race never happened.

To be sure, there were some high points. I broke four minutes in the mile, got loads of press and my story began making the rounds at every major shoe company. But it wasn't enough. To this day I still don't know what the people in the running world want. I'm not asking for something that my peers don't have.

But all that pressure did slowly build up in me. The 15- or 19-year-old Brandon would have welcomed the challenge and used it as fuel, but not the 26-to-29-year-old Brandon. He couldn't handle the burden. It became a bad source of stress, and I tried every conceivable way to funnel that energy into positive thoughts, but it never sustained.

When you stand on the starting line of a race, it's almost like a fighter standing in the center of the ring. You have to have the confidence that the work you've put in will allow you to win the fight. I was fighting too many inner battles to be prepared to stand on the starting line with the sole goal of winning.

So often during those years I embraced the inner bitch and found myself taking the easy way out. I gave myself excuse after excuse, but it always came back to the fact that I was working too much, too stressed out, had too many factors working against me, and not enough time to be a real athlete. I tried to not let those creep in--and a few times in there I was able to defeat that inner bitch--but more and more that inner bitch was winning and I didn't like it.

Even if it didn't show on the outside or come up in conversations, I was often jealous and angry at opportunities, like endorsements, that my competitors had been given. It's no secret that this kind of emotional response is neither healthy nor conducive to success. But my way of thinking was this: After all the years I'd spent training and all the sacrifices I'd made, I had earned the right to be a full-time professional athlete and to enjoy all the benefits afforded by that status. But, man, I could just not get lucky enough. And in time, all that jealousy and anger led to bitterness. I was only in my late 20s, but I was becoming a bitter and resentful old man.

Things finally reached a breaking point in May 2016.

Quitting My Job to Pursue My Dreams

Nearly every day for three years, I had the dream of going in to work and quitting my job. Well, guess what? I finally did.

Talk about taking a chance. At that point, my hand was finally forced. Or, just maybe, I was attempting to write this book from behind that green desk at work instead of the comfort of my home. In any event, when my work schedule was posted for June of that year, one thing stood out like a sore big toe: I didn't get the days off that I needed so that I could race and, hopefully, qualify for the Olympic Trials.

This placed me at a crossroads. In reality this situation should have come up much earlier, but because I had been embracing the "risk" of quitting, my inner bitch allowed me to experience comfort. Comfort is nice. Even depression, sadness, stress, and excuses can eventually become comfortable. And that's exactly where I found myself. And I had to decide, at that specific point in time, whether to stay at my job and have my lifelong goal of running in the Olympic Trials come down to one opportunity to qualify, or quit my job and have the extra time to participate in the three races I might need.

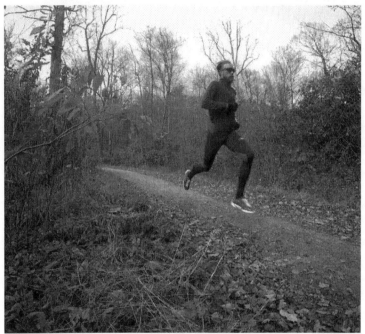

While work might not have always been fun, it was always worth it to be able to train in my favorite place on planet Earth (photo by Bill Wilde)

One thing I have to explain here is the complexity of the qualifying process for the Olympic Trials. The rules are created by our governing body, United States of America Track and Field (USATF), and all athletes need to abide by them. In 2016 the rules stated that a runner must run 1,500 meters in 3:38 or faster to be guaranteed a spot on the starting line. Now, if 30 declared athletes didn't run under 3:38, the organizers would follow a descending-order list based on time, until they reached 30 athletes.

The window for qualifying was extremely short, literally just one week before the start of the Trials. And to make it even more complicated, athletes didn't have to declare in the 1500-meter run until almost halfway through the ten-day Olympic Trials event. This allowed some athletes to keep their name on the list and run their primary event first. If they bombed out, they could run the 1500-meters as a backup.

On June 4th, one week after quitting my guest services job, I ran 3:38.20 at the Furman Elite 1500-meter race in Greenville, SC. At that point I was somewhere around 15th overall on that descending order list. Which was both good and bad. With three weeks left to qualify, 15 more athletes would have to jump me, but without an official qualifying time, I was nervous with each and every meet that was contested until the window closed.

I wanted to not pay attention to the other races because they were out of my hands, but I don't operate like that. And I needed to know. So I found myself sitting up late stalking race results and live feeds to watch meets that were on the west coast, just to see if anyone would hop me. The first weekend went by with a breeze. Torrential downpours prevented fast times at a meet in Portland, OR, where some of the best runners in the nation were chasing times. Then, with just two weeks to go, some people got hungry and greedy and were often stuck chasing times and had to make concessions in training to be ready to race again just a few days later.

All of this played into my hands as we entered the final days before the trials. I ran one more race in the middle of June to try and lower my mark and guarantee myself a spot in the trials, but I made some mistakes early in that race, then tried too hard to make up ground and found myself out of fight and energy during the final 400 meters of the race. This led to what I believe was one of my worst performances of 2016 with a time of 3:40.1 at the Princeton Last Chance Qualifier.

That was a testament to how far my training and fitness had come in one year. Had I run that race and time a year earlier, it would've been a personal record time by 2 seconds but now it was considered a failure. That's what's so remarkable about lowering your personal record time; it opens your mind to new possibilities and new normals. Times above 3:40 were now considered bad performances and I loved it.

Anyway, after suffering through the final two weeks of watching people chase times, I entered the qualifying trials for a possible spot on the U. S. Olympics Team with the 18th-ranked time during the qualifying window, and was guaranteed a spot on the starting line. I finally realized the first step in my dream of qualifying for the Olympic Trials.

Now, back to quitting my job. As you can now see, the process of qualifying for the Olympic Trials can be a bit tedious, and I knew that I might need more than one opportunity to get my qualifying mark. I watched as some runners' opportunities were ruined by rain and other weather-related issues during the month of June, and had I not quit, I would have been in that same boat myself. Races and conditions can be unpredictable, and any of my opportunities could have been ruined by any number of unplanned incidents a fall, weather, bad pacing, a stomach bug, travel complications, or some other personal disaster. You name it, I've seen it.

With that thought in my head, my work schedule in my hand and only one opportunity to race, I was at the crossroads I had dreamed about for three years. On one hand I was jumping for joy. I was exhilarated to finally have the reason (or excuse) I needed to quit my job. On the other hand, though, I also experienced a strong degree of insecurity. Quitting my job meant I would be totally, completely, unequivocally, 100 percent on my own. There would be no more biweekly pay checks or health insurance coverage associated with a job. It would now be up to me to race and hustle to make ends meet.

Of course I also knew that all I needed was one big performance to give me that elusive running contract I so desired. As you might imagine, my emotions were all over the place for about three days as I tried hard not to make a rash decision. I thought about it, talked with my parents, girlfriend, and best friend, and thought about it some more. After several days of deliberation, we all came to the same conclusion: it had reached the point where my job had interfered for long enough, and there was no question that had I to choose the pursuit of my dream over the comfort of a paycheck.

Today, I completely understand my former employer's position. I really do. I was contracted to work, and they needed me for those dates. And during the past few years I missed several meets because I needed to stay and work.

But this wasn't the same at all. Those weren't qualifying meets for the Olympic Trials.

So our arrangement had finally expired and I had to take back control of my life and empower myself. Over those few days of contemplation, I realized that I hadn't really been all-in on my dream. I was using too many things as crutches and, as a result, had remained unempowered. By finally making the decision to quit my job and walking into my boss's office and doing it, I was kicking the inner bitch out of my head and empowering myself again.

This wasn't a risk. To many on the outside it looked like I was jumping head first off a cliff into murky water, but to me I was sliding into a nice warm jacuzzi. I do hate that it came down to me providing only five days notice before leaving, but that was the circumstance. There were some fun times and I made some dear friends while working there, and for the most part of those three years, my bosses and coworkers had been incredibly understanding and flexible with my racing schedule. But it all ran its course and it was time for me to be "BHudg" full time. No more dressing up, putting on a tie and a smile and faking my way through an eight-hour shift. I now had the power to chase my dream uninhibited.

Boy, did it pay off. I don't think it's a coincidence that my best performance of the year came just one week after quitting that job. At that meet, I was light on my feet and light in spirit. I was finally happy to be chasing my dream. It also made my decision look less "risky" to those around me. It proved to them that what I knew inside was real. I was meant to do this and I could do this.

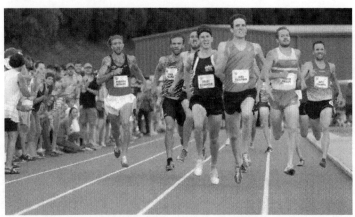

Flying by Ford Palmer on the outside! Kicking down the homestretch to my Olympic Trials qualifying time of 3:38.20. (photo courtesy of scrunners.com)

Kicking the Inner Bitch

Embracing the inner bitch of comfort can be very, very rewarding. As hokey as it may sound, at times it's almost like how people describe the high associated with heroin. A nice warm blanket dulls the edges of the world and takes certain stress off your chest. As you now know, I have lost the battle with my inner bitch more times than I would care to admit, but there are also a ton of times I can tell you that I kicked that inner bitch out and went on with the goal for that day.

Defeating the inner bitch is not an overnight process. It's ultimately what gives you the tools for dedication to your desire. Realize that you are going to lose some of those battles. In the beginning you may even lose a lot of them. But you have to keep swinging at that bitch and, in time, you will start to win more of those battles than you lose. That inner bitch of self-doubt wants to keep you warm and comfortable. Knocking him or her in the teeth will empower you. Prime examples of conquering the inner bitch and punching him or her in the face can include getting out to do a workout when you don't want to . . . introducing yourself to someone to whom you have been afraid to talk . . . eating something new that scares you, but that you know is healthy . . . admitting a fault . . . or embracing a challenge. There are tons of chances to start to win over the inner bitch. Try to harness the feeling of accomplishment after each success and get some momentum going.

These little wins won't be visible to most people, but they will motivate and encourage you. These are the foundation to your success; taking steps that often look like risk to outsiders. Just as not much had changed for me during three years of working as a guest services representative, I had little victory after little victory of beating the inner bitch. So when I finally had to haul off and punch the inner bitch in the face, I was able to do that and move on to my next mission. So, keep swinging and tallying up those little victories. They give you the confidence to take that big step. Oh, and guess what: when you get to the other side, there is a new bigger and badder inner bitch that you are going to have to take on, so get ready...

Standing on the Starting Line

Standing on the starting line at Hayward Field on the University of Oregon's campus at the 2016 U.S. Olympic Track and Field Trials is the most mind-boggling thing I have ever experienced. Somehow, this experience was even tougher for me than dealing with the physical battles of my vasculitis, the emotional battles of anxiety and depression or any fight I've had with my girlfriend.

Which sucked. The Olympic experience was supposed to be one of the most joyful and satisfying moments in my life. This was supposed to be my moment of triumph over everything that life had thrown at me. But there I was, standing on the starting line of the biggest race of my life,

103

simultaneously trying to control my nerves, focus on the task at hand and not shit myself, and I realized deep down that I wasn't prepared for this. I've been dreaming about this opportunity since I was 13 years old. This was supposed to be what I wanted, but once I was in that moment I thought I craved so much, I wished I could've been somewhere hiding.

It wasn't the fun experience I imagined it would be which, looking back, explains ultimately why I failed. It wasn't a lack of fitness, nor was it a lack of speed. It was a lack of fun. I had embraced the little inner bitch of doubt and nerves. I hadn't given my personal best that day. The stress had caught me, and it kicked my ass. I never could have imagined as a 13-year-old the significance and weight that getting to this starting line would have on my life and on the lives of those following my journey. No amount of racing or imagery could've prepared me for the weight of the situation I found myself in on July 7th, 2016. I had trained for this and dreamed about this for so long, but had no clue about how to handle myself on this stage. I tried to act like this was business as usual for me, but on the inside I was filled with the doubt and anxiety that would eventually cripple my chances of achieving my goal of making the final round of 12 and finishing in the top 10.

Now as I suffer through another relapse with my Vasculitis in 2017, I have the daunting task of conquering not just Vasculitis again, but many of the same obstacles that I faced in the previous three years leading into the Olympic Trials in 2016. I handled the Olympic Trials so poorly emotionally in 2016 that I feel like I owe it to myself, my family, and my fans to go back and conquer the inner bitch of doubt and nerves. I want to show the world I belong on that stage and can do so while having fun this time. It will be a tall task physically. I'll be 33 in 2020, long past what most consider the prime for middle distance runners. But I don't care. I've beat worse odds before in my life. If I get back there and bow out again in the semi-final, but it was my personal best that day and I enjoy myself while I'm there, then it will be a true dream come true. Maybe then I can finally hang up my racing spikes and start the next chapter of my life without any regrets.

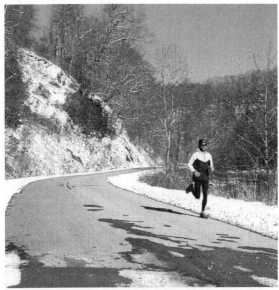

It's easy for the inner bitch to win on days like this (photo by Bill Wilde)

Walking Through Hell for Happiness

Life doesn't care how much knowledge and experience you have gained. For some people life just isn't going to be easy. It's going to beat you down. And if you let it, it can very easily pin you there. So those of us who have it rough in life need to find ways to get past it and move on. We need to realize that it's not our fault; it's just the hand that life has dealt us. If we allow it to, it can ruin all sorts of things, from our relationships to even our chances to be successful.

If this describes your life situation (as it does mine), here's a tip: don't get mad, get even.

It's easy to get angry when we see our friends and family members seem to skirt through life without a care in the world. Believe me, I know. Well, news flash, that's just not going to be you. I often compare life to a poker game, one in which we're stuck with the hand we're dealt. We have to figure out a way to play that hand. It might sound rough and a bit insensitive, but trust me—experience tells me that if you dwell on it, the pain and self-wallow is only going to get worse. So what the hell do you do then when life deals you a shitty card?

One of the questions people often ask me is "How?" They wonder how I've fought through so many different obstacles in life and yet continue to chase my dreams. The short answer is craziness. The long answer is baby steps.

Sometimes when I look back, I truly don't know how I have done it time and time again. But each time, I slowly dragged myself up off the mat, got my gloves up in front of my face and started swinging again. Just like a boxer who has been pummeled to the ground, I often get up foggy, staggering and searching for the ropes to help me up. When you hit rock bottom on numerous occasions, it can become an easy place to stay. Believe it or not, being depressed and sad can be comfortable because you know what to expect. You begin to find comfort in your self-pity. It's a dangerous slope, but it allows you to have an excuse for everything.

As I said earlier, getting up is the hard part, but once you're up, you'd better get your hands up and steady your feet because life won't hold its punches. This is important, so I'll say it again: before you worry about fighting back, get up and steady yourself. Once you create the right mindset, getting up can become second nature. Now, that doesn't mean that you're going to pop right back up every time you get knocked down. In fact, there will be times when you have to use your full 10 count to get back up. Or, hell, you might even occasionally get saved by the bell. Our circumstances and experiences in life define us as people. Those circumstances and experiences can also become an excuse for success or failure. What you choose to do with your circumstances and experiences is up to you.

So how do we get back up? How do we learn to do what seems impossible? I truly believe that the first step is acknowledging that the situation or experience that has knocked you down sucks. Own it. It's fine to hurt, cry and even stay in bed sometimes. it's normal to want to hide or put up a facade when things happen. You just have to own it and realize that it's all temporary and part of the process. This process isn't a day, a week or even a month long. In fact, for some it will be a lifelong battle. So learn to fall and learn that it's okay to cower in and shut off. We need those moments of weakness and despair to grow.

It's taken me months (and even years, at times) to learn and grow from my tragic moments. But own it and accept that you can't deny it or hide from it. That will only make the problem worse. Own it and realize that you're going to have to walk through hell to get back on top—but be okay with that. When you are at the bottom of a giant mountain staring up at the peak, the top seems so far away. And that first step toward the mountain is the most important and the hardest to take. Take one step, then another, then another, then another, and before you know it you will find yourself well on the way to the top.

To give you an idea of how desperate and dark things have become for me at times, here are a few lyrics of poetry (or music) that I wrote down. They show you just how far gone my own mind can get.

Do you know what it's like to not be able to live in
your own head?
Your thoughts are corrupt and I don't trust yourself
I'm stuck in a living hell, I mine as well be dead
There's a monster inside, who has eaten my wealth

I've admitted defeat
From all that I seek
The devil has breathed
Life inside of me

Obviously, these are uplifting words! But they tell a very surreal story of where my headspace was during these times. Don't be afraid to write down your unfiltered thoughts. They are for you and no one else unless you choose to share them. If you want, they can remain locked away as a little reminder of where you have been. Raw emotions can create beautiful art that can be enjoyed for years to come. Many or even all of the words you write might never see the light of day, but they do have the potential to paint a vivid picture of a time in your life that will become important to you years from now. So cherish these moments for what they are: the absolute rock-bottom and a chance to grow.

When I arrived in Boone, NC, I was an absolute walking disaster and in desperate need of some relief from life, and this tiny town hidden in the Blue Ridge Mountains came to my rescue. I will forever be indebted to my friends who helped make that possible (Brian Graves, Chris Moen, Sody, and Mark Sullivan). Graves found me a job working at

Westglow Resort and Spa and the boys let me sleep on the couch and share rooms while I gathered some cash and slowly pieced my life together over the summer of 2013. For almost a year, Moen had not just been living with me, but sharing a room with me! Wow!

No matter your current situation, you have to fight to find your happiness. It is sometimes impossible for that happiness to even remain in the same places and come from the same things. You have to listen, learn, grow, and search to find your happy place. I am warning you though: it's difficult to find, but that doesn't mean that you should shy away. Learn to find happiness in chasing and pursuing dreams and goals. In fact, when you are chasing your goals you might find yourself sitting in your own personal hell. If so, that means you are probably on the right path! It means that your journey is worth something, that your goals matter to you and that your life has passion and meaning. You may have failed, so what? The real happiness comes from continuing chase it through hell regardless of the outcome or possibility of failure!

Fight Like Hell

I've offered you stories from my process that got me to the starting line of my dream. How did I ultimately complete my hero's journey that Moen alluded to in the foreword? Just like all heroes, I approached my inmost cave completely unprepared, but when I emerged I had the courage to embrace the challenge. With a stable support system under me, I had the freedom to fight as I needed.

I found my desire in that inmost cave and let that desire drive my motivation every single day. This is the solution for dealing with almost any adversity in life. Anyone who has had an extreme desire or passion in life will tell you that the true secret is finding your desire. It gets much easier when your work and passion fulfills your inner most desires. Just like eating that chocolate treat or drinking that cold beer on a hot day, your work can stimulate that same reward pathway in your brain if you allow it. It sounds romantic, but as I've alluded to throughout the book, it's often ugly. It won't be easy going through the trials of your ordeal, but as long as you keep you remind yourself of your desire when things get tough, your actions will take care of themselves.

Numerous times in my life, I remember lying in bed while hooked up to countless IVs to save my life and thinking to myself, "Once I get out of this bed, I'll be damned if I'm going to let this thing beat me." While I never completely understand the struggles that lie ahead, once I was free of the IVs then it was one foot in front of the other. Once you are out of the bed or your inmost cave, you can't look back. The race or challenge is always in front of you. Focus on the day that you have. Running itself is difficult physically and mentally, but having a coach and a training plan makes the path clear to follow each and every day.

Lots of books and research focus on the power of positive thinking. And while I totally agree with most of it, you also have to remember that I am a realist. I believe in science and I know that sometimes, no matter how positively you think, there are certain things that just can't be overcome. I do, however, believe that there are situations where a positive mindset and outlook can be beneficial. In my case, with GPA, I knew I was physically able to handle activity again; it would just require a lot of mental fortitude to get back out there and get back to a level that I thought was successful. With an incurable disease that can comeback at any point without warning, if reminds me of one of my favorite Star Wars quotes from Han Solo. Han tells C3PO, a protocol and etiquette droid that often assess the risk of certain situations, "Don't ever tell me the odds."

When you have the answer to why, all you have to do is figure out how. Believe it or not, that's the easy part. If your goals seem unattainable and you focus too much on the odds you may have to overcome, then you will never get the how. My approach is to first set a big goal, then list each of the steps that will be required to achieve it.

That's how you fight. You have to find something you love—something that, if you don't do it, you can't live with yourself. For me that was chasing the professional running dream. For others, maybe that's writing a book, starting a business, becoming an actor, starting a band, becoming a teacher, learning to surf, or doing something that has a positive impact on your community. The list is really endless. While your circumstances may dictate how you chase your dream, to hell with them, create your opportunities for happiness!

As a distance runner, my goal since age 13 was to break the four-minute mile and become a professional distance runner. I was inspired in 2001 by watching Alan Webb set the national high school record for the mile in 3:53.43. At that moment I became obsessed with the idea of joining the sub 4 minute mile club. I had been running for three years at that point and I now I had my mission. At times that goal seemed very close, and at other times it seemed impossible. My original goal was to do it in high school, but it didn't happen. I worked toward the same goal when I was in college. Then I got sick, and I wondered if I'd ever even be able to get back to running, but I never lost the desire to join the sub 4 minute club. No matter how far away that goal seemed, it was always something that I wanted to accomplish.

I wish the dream would've come true during my first comeback at age 23. This story would've been much easier to tell, but that didn't happen. As it turned out, I had much more fighting to do. I had to go through several different incarnations of myself before I was ready for the final fight. Finally, at 28 years old, I checked off my first goal and used that momentum to complete my journey. This was something I set out to do at age 13, and while I may have lost my way several times, it was one thing I really wanted. When you have your thing, fighting becomes much easier. The "how" answers itself. You do what is necessary so you can do what you love. That meant fifteen years of suffering through my test, fighting my enemies of self doubt, exploring my inmost cave, and finally completing my journey.

Now, looking back, I realize how truly lucky I am to be able to run again with a vasculitis disorder. So many people who suffer from vasculitis disorders struggle to do simple, mundane daily activities, much less reach the highest level of endurance sports. If I had focused on all the negatives along the way, I never would've made it. Now go out and find your inspiration to go the distance in your own life.

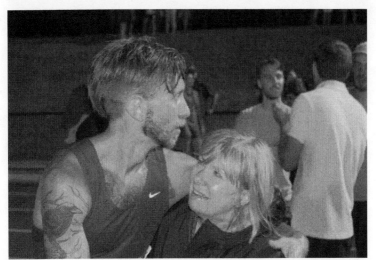

That moment when all your trials and tribulations were worth it!
(photo by Tim Meigs)

About the Authors:

Brandon Hudgins
Brandon has been active as a long-distance runner since he began competing in the sport at age 10. After being diagnosed with vasculitis in 2008, he continued to run, and in the past several years has achieved elite status in the sport. He completed a BA in Physical Education: Fitness and Wellness at Winthrop University in 2009 and finished his MS in Exercise Science: Strength and Conditioning from Appalachian State University in 2011. His thesis in graduate school resulted in a published article in the Journal of Strength and Conditioning Research. On August 7, 2015, Brandon became the 448th American to run a mile in less than 4-minutes, when he completed the Sir Walter Raleigh Miler in 3:59.67. He lives in Jamestown, North Carolina, where he continues to chase his dream of Olympic Glory. His days are filled with training, being a personal running coach, and working closely with the Vasculitis Foundation as their Health Ambassador. For more about Brandon and his journey visit www.BrandonHudgins.com

John Fries
John is a writer, graphic designer, digital media producer, and principal at Fries Communications, a marketing, communications and media consultancy and creative studio. He is honored to work with the Vasculitis Foundation and Team Brandon. To see more of John's work visit his website www.johnfries.com

The Vasculitis Foundation
The Foundation established Team Brandon in March 2016 to support Brandon as he trained for the 2016 Summer Olympics. Although he didn't make the

Olympic Team, Brandon's amazing spirit and positive outlook on life inspired more than 300 team members to participate in weekly exercise challenges to become more active and healthy. Members also participated in awareness challenges issued by Brandon. In 2017, VF Team Brandon continues to help even more patients living with vasculitis and their family members achieve their own personal best. Brandon's personal experience as a patient and his educational background gives him a unique perspective and understanding on motivating patients living with chronic illnesses. He continues to promote health and wellness as part of his ambassador role with the Vasculitis Foundation.

To donate, learn more about Brandon's role with VF, or join Team Brandon, visit:

http://www.vasculitisfoundation.org/

Made in the USA
Columbia, SC
31 May 2018